Terminology &
Communication Skills
in the Health Sciences

Terminology & Communication Skills in the Health Sciences

Office of Medical Studies
University of North Carolina-Chapel Hill

Reston Publishing Company, Inc.
Reston, Virginia 22090
A Prentice-Hall Company

Library of Congress Cataloging in Publication Data

Lea, James, 1941-
    Terminology and communication skills in the health
sciences.

    1. Medicine—Terminology—Programmed instruction.
2. Medical libraries—Programmed instruction. 3. Eng-
lish language—Programmed instruction. I. Title.
[DNLM: 1. Communication. 2. Medicine. 3. Nomencla-
ture. WZ345 L433t]
R123.L38   610'.1'4   74-34304
ISBN 0-87909-822-8
ISBN 0-87909-821-X pbk.

© *1975 by Reston Publishing Company, Inc.*

A Prentice-Hall Company   Reston, Virginia 22090

10 9 8 7 6 5 4 3   Printed in the United States of America

Table of Contents

INTRODUCTION, vii

SECTION ONE
Elements of Health Sciences Terminology, 1
Introduction, 3

Unit 1, 5
    Review List, 11
Unit 2, 13
    Review List, 17
Review Test for Units 1 & 2, 19
    Answers: Units 1 & 2, 20

Unit 3, 21
    Review List, 26
Unit 4, 27
    Review List, 32
Review Test for Units 3 & 4, 33
    Answers: Units 3 & 4, 34

Unit 5, 37
    Review List, 42
Unit 6, 43
    Review List, 48
Review Test for Units 5 & 6, 49
    Answers: Units 5 & 6, 50

Unit 7, 51
    Review List, 56
Unit 8, 57
    Review List, 62
Review Test for Units 7 & 8, 63
    Answers: Units 7 & 8, 65

Unit 9, 67
    Review List, 72

Unit 10, 73
 Review List, 78
Review Test for Units 9 & 10, 79
 Answers: Units 9 & 10, 80

SECTION TWO
Using the Health Sciences Library, 81
 Introduction, 83

Pre-Test: Library Unit 1, 85
 Pre-Test Answers, 86
Unit 1, 87
Review Test for Unit 1, 107
 Answers: Unit 1, 108

Pre-Test: Library Unit 2, 111
 Pre-Test Answers, 111
Unit 2, 113
Review Test for Unit 2, 119
 Answers: Unit 2, 120

SECTION THREE
Organization and Expression for the Health Professional, 121
 Introduction, 123

Pre-Test: Organization Unit 1, 125
 Pre-Test Answers, 125
Unit 1, 127
Review Test for Unit 1, 133
 Answers: Unit 1, 134

Pre-Test: Organization Unit 2, 135
 Pre-Test Answers, 136
Unit 2, 137

Pre-Test: Organization Unit 3, 145
 Pre-Test Answers, 145
Unit 3, 147

Introduction

TO THE STUDENT:

This self-instructional program in *Terminology and Communication Skills in Health Sciences* has been prepared to give you practice in using some of the skills and techniques that you will need throughout your health professional training. The contents of the program have been selected by faculty members in schools of dentistry, medicine, medical technology, nursing, pharmacy, and public health. Most of the practice exercises and projects included in this program are samples of actual professional school study activities. So whatever your chosen field in health science, you should find this program of value.

Now a few words about how this program is put together and how you should use it. The term *self-instructional* means that as you use these materials you are instructing yourself. The program offers you material to be learned, opportunities to practice using what you are learning, and means by which you can check your own learning progress. But *you* are in charge of putting the program to use. You are doing the instructing.

The new material—the *input*—in this program is broken into small blocks. It's more manageable that way. After each small block of input, you will have an opportunity to *practice* using the new material by answering a question or solving a problem. Then immediately after you practice, you will get *feedback*. The feedback will tell you how you should have answered the question or solved the problem; it will let you check how well you are learning. You don't have to wait until the next class meeting to find out!

Unit 1 in the health sciences terminology series is designed to introduce you to self-instructional learning. As you work through it, you will discover that this form of learning allows some privileges and makes some demands:

1: You may *work at your own pace*, taking what time you need to learn from each unit. You may also be able to work through any unit as many times as you need to.
2: You must *work honestly* by not looking ahead and by not checking the feedback until you have made a genuine effort to supply an answer yourself.
3: You must *work steadily* and not allow yourself to fall behind schedule in completing the assigned number of units each term.

If you begin your work in this self-instructional program with a commitment to these basic self-regulations, you will find that

1: You will *learn more material.*
2: You will *learn faster and more enjoyably.*
3: You will *retain what you learn.*

Remember that this self-instructional program has been designed to benefit *you* as a health science student. If your use of it is to be an effective and enjoyable learning experience, you must accept the personal responsibility for (1) working through each unit honestly and conscientiously and (2) scheduling your work so that you can complete the program in the time allotted for it. Don't forget—*you* are the self-instructor, so *you* must accept the instructional responsibilities.

*   *   *

You might be interested to know that many people have contributed in numerous ways to the development of this program. Some of the names on the long list are Merrel Flair, Hugh Burford, Clif Crandall, Dorothy Long, Carol Fray, and B.H. Kaplan, of the University of North Carolina; Rita and Stuart Johnson, of the Health Sciences Consortium; some 600 health sciences students all over the United States, who patiently explained to me what was good and what was bad about earlier versions of these units; and Diane Lea, who supplied excellent research support and who just generally makes life a lot easier.

For invaluable editorial assistance, great patience, and general help in getting these materials into your hands, David Ungerer and Don Hardy of Reston Publishing Company deserve much credit.

And a special word needs to be said to the North Carolina Health Manpower Development Program, which supported the writing of a prototype of this program several years ago. The special word is, thanks!

*   *   *

I would be delighted to have you join the people who have contributed to this program. Please send me whatever suggestions for its improvement you may have.

JAMES LEA

Chapel Hill,
North Carolina

Section One

Elements of Health Sciences Terminology

Introduction

You are about to begin work on a 10-unit program in Health Sciences Terminology. In this program you will acquire a basic vocabulary of terms that are used in many health professional disciplines. In the process of learning this system, you will practice building words from word parts and recognizing a wide range of word-part meanings. More important, perhaps, you will learn the system by which health professional terminology works.

Objectives:
   When you complete this self-instructional program, you should be able to

   1: Recognize, define, and use correctly a basic, multidisciplinary health sciences vocabulary in sentences that deal with anatomy, disease, and other health topics.
   2: Translate a long paragraph of complex professional terminology into layman's terms.

   In addition, I hope that you complete this program with satisfaction and confidence in your new ability to use the language of a health professional.

Components:
   The program has two components. Your instructor may not assign all of them, but be certain that you have those that are required before you begin work on any part of the program.

   1: Ten self-instructional Units.
   2: Five Review Tests, one following each two self-instructional Units.

You should also have a good medical dictionary at hand to help with tricky definitions or for general review. I recommend *Taber's Cyclopedic Medical Dictionary*, 12th edition.

Taber's is published by F. A. Davis, Inc., Philadelphia, and you can buy it for about $9.50.

Cut a heavy piece of paper to use as a cover card. This card is to be placed over the left-hand margin of each page of self-instructional material in this program.

UNIT 1

1: In these self-instructional units on professional terminology, you will be working with short sequences of input, practice, and feedback. All blocks of new information are called *input*. In fact, all the information in this sequence is

input
input .

2: Following each piece of new information, you will encounter a blank that you are expected to fill in. This is a *practice* opportunity, a very important part of the learning process. Whenever you encounter a blank, use the op-

practice
portunity to *practice* with new information by filling it in.

3: Some practice opportunities in these units will ask you to *recall* new information that you have just received. At other times, you will use new information to solve a *problem* or make a judgment about a term's meaning. In other

recalling
problem
words, practice can be either *recalling* new information or *problem* solving.

4: Regardless of what kind of practice you are asked to do, you will receive *feedback*—the correct answer—immediately after each practice. So as soon as you fill in each practice blank, you should slide down the cover card

feedback
to receive the correct answer, called *feedback*.

5: If you make an error in practice, that's all right, because that's what practice is for. Whenever your answer does not agree with the feedback, look back at the input to find out where you went wrong; then *correct* your practice

correct

answer. If real learning is to occur, it is important that you *correct* any incorrect practice answers.

6: Some practice opportunities will require only *one* word for a correct answer. Others will require *two or more* words. You will have to make your own judgment as to whether a particular blank should be filled in with *one* word or with *two* words.

one
two or more

7: Because the input, practice, and feedback in these self-instructional units are arranged in a progressive sequence, you should not *look ahead* before completing the practice frame you are working on. You may look back over completed work, but you should never *look ahead*.

look ahead

8: Here's a chance to review this brief introduction working with the self-instructional terminology units:

Each learning step in these units consists of *input*, *feedback*, and *practice*. An error should be *corrected*. The success of your effort depends largely upon taking advantage of every opportunity to *practice* with new information.

input
practice, feedback
corrected

practice

9: Health sciences fields all have large vocabularies, but many of them have several *word parts* in common. You can achieve a command of a great number of words by learning a relatively few *word* parts.

word

10: In language studies, such as this one, a *root* is the word base to which other word parts are attached. *Hale* is the *root* of the words *in/hale* and *ex/hale*.

root

11: In the terms *hyper/tension* and *hypo/tension*, the root is *tension*.

tension

12: In question 11, the same root is combined with two different *prefixes* to produce two different terms. The prefixes in question 11 are *hyper* and *hypo*.

hyper, hypo
prefix

13: In the term *hyposensitive* the word part *hypo* is a *prefix* meaning "abnormally decreased," or "deficient." A hyposensitive microorganism is *deficient* in sensitivity.

deficient

14: As you might expect, the prefix *hyper-* means "abnormally increased" or "excessive." A microorganism that exhibits abnormally high sensitivity would be described as *hyper*/sensitive.

hyper

15: If the term *plasminemia* refers to plasmin in the circulating blood, build a word that describes a condition of excessive plasmin in the circulating blood *hyper/plasminemia*.

hyper/plasminemia

16: Here's a problem. In the word that you built in question 15, which word element means "a condition of the blood"? (Think!) *emia*

emia

17: To get the correct answer in question 16, you did something that you'll have to do often in learning and using professional terminology: you found the two word parts that you knew and made a good judgment about the meaning of the unfamiliar word part. This mental activity might be called *terminology problem solving*. Throughout your mental health training, you will frequently engage in *Terminology problem solving*.

terminology
  problem solving

18: Another means of building health science terms from different word parts is the use of the *combining form*, which is a vowel added to a root. *Electr/o* is a combining form. In the words end/o/scope and end/o/blast, end/o is the *Combining form*

combining form

19: During your health professional training, you will often encounter the word element *fibr-*, which means "fibrous" or "fiber." Create a combining form of this word element and add it to another word element that means "giving rise to" or "causing"; you will build a new term meaning "causing the development of fibers." *fibr o* /genic

fibr/o

(Now you're beginning to work with professional terms.)

20: *Endoscope* is a term built from a combining form and a word. In the term end/o/scope
    end/o is the *Combining form*
    scope is the *Word*

combining form
word

21: The meaning and usages of terms change as their endings change. When the -e ending of end/o/scop/e changes to a -y ending, the new term means "visual examination of interior structures of the body with an endoscope." Notice that *scop* now appears as a root. In the word end/o/-scop/y,
    end/o is the *Combining form*
    scop is the *root*
    -y is the *ending*

combining form
root
ending

22: *End/o/scop/e* and *end/o/scop/y* are both nouns. You can build the adjective form of the term by using an -ic ending. Build a term that is an adjective referring to the use of an endoscope or endoscopy *endoscopic* *end/o/scop/ic*

end/o/scop/ic

end/o

23: An *end/o/crine* gland is one that secretes internally. Look back at questions 21 and 22 and decide which part of the term end/o/crine means "within," "inward," or "internal." *end o*

ect/o/scop/y

24: The combining form *ect/o* means "external" or "outside." Using word parts with which you have just become familiar, build a term (a noun) that means "external inspection of an organ." *ect o scop y*

(If you got that one correct, you're doing a good job!)

etc/o/derm
end/o/derm/ic

25: The word elements *derm* and *derma* refer to skin. Build a noun that means, "the outermost layer of skin or cells." *ect o derm* Now build an adjective that refers to "an internal layer of skin or cells." *en tro derm ic*

26: If you found question 25 a little tricky, don't worry. You will learn the correct forms of some health sciences terms only through experience in using them. For example, you'll find that the adjective ending -al is used in a simple term that means "pertaining to the true skin." What do you think the term is? *derm al*

derm/al

prefix
combining form
root
ending

27: Now try this one. In the term *en/cephal/o/dyn/ic*,
en is the *prefix*
cephal/o is a *combining form*
dyn looks like a *root*
ic is the *ending*

end/o/gen/ic

28: In question 19, you used the word element *-gen/ic*, which means "giving rise to" or "causing." Try building a word that means "caused internally." (Think about terms that you have been using.) *end o gen ic*

bio/gen/ic

29: If *bio* is a word element meaning "life" or "living," can you build a word that means "causing or giving rise to a living organism"? *bio gen ic*

30: You have already learned that endoscopy is the visual examination of interior structures of the body by use of an endoscope. Now think for a moment, and then build a word that would mean "examination of a body (using an instrument) for the presence or absence of life." *bio scop y*

bio/scop/

(That may have been difficult, even with the clue. But if you got it correct, or came close, you are doing good work.)

31: The adjective ending *-ic* frequently changes to *-tic* when it follows a vowel. So we have bio/tic, meaning "pertaining to living organisms." If the prefix *anti-* means "counteracting" or "effective against," what is the meaning of anti/bio/tic? *active against a living organism*

counteracting, or
  effective against
  living organisms

32: A chemical substance that is administered to counteract certain living organisms (which are presumed to be harmful to the human body) is called an *antibiotic* substance.

anti/bio/tic

33: Call upon word elements that you have learned previously in this unit to build a word to describe a substance that is effective against life-causing agents *antibiogenic*

anti/bio/gen/ic

34: Antibiotic (in question 32) can be used as either an adjective—you've already noticed the -ic adjective ending— or a noun. The same is true for many words that end in -ic. So a chemical compound that counteracts certain living organisms is not only described as an *antibiotic*, it is also named *antibiotic*.

anti/bio/tic
anti/bio/tic

35: The word *febrile* means "pertaining to fever" or "feverish." A chemical compound administered to counteract fever is called an *antifebrile* compound.

anti/febrile

36: A condition of high blood pressure with associated feverishness might be called _*febrile*_ hyper/tension.

febrile

37: In the term *febrile hyper/tension,*
hyper means _*abnormally increased*_
febrile means _*feverish*_
tension refers to _*blood pressure*_

abnormally increased
feverish
blood pressure

(If you got those correct, you did a good job of terminology problem solving.)

38: The word element *somat/o* means "the body." A general professional term that means "treatment aimed at relieving or curing ills of the body" would be *somato*/therapy.

somat/o

39: When you see a word that has the root *somat*, the word probably refers to the entire body. *Somat/o/metr/y*, for example, means "measurement of the _*entire*_ _*body*_."

entire
body

40: Use a word element that you learned earlier in this unit to build a word meaning "examination (using an instrument) somat/o/scop/y

somat

	of the entire body." _somat scop y_ (handwritten)
	41: Now put together a familiar word that refers to "the interrelations of body and mind." psych/o/*somat*/ic
	42: The word element *ser/o* may refer either to the clear, watery fluids that coat membrane surfaces or to the watery component of blood. The most common noun that uses this word element is *serum*. What word would you build to mean "diagnostic visual examination (using an instrument) of serum"? *ser o scop*/y

ser/o/scop

	43: *Serum* or *serum derivatives* are often used to treat certain diseases or disorders. Use a word element that you have used before in this unit to build a word to mean "treatment using serum." *ser o therapy*

ser/o/therapy

ser/o/toxin

	44: A *toxin* is a substance that is poisonous to organisms. A toxin existing in the blood serum is a *ser o toxin*

anti/toxin

	45: An agent that is effective against toxins is called an *anti toxin*

(See how quickly you recalled that one?)

	46: The word element upon which *toxin* is based is toxic/o. Use a word element that you have already learned to build a word meaning "causing or giving rise to poisons."

toxic/o/gen/ic

toxic o gen ic (handwritten)

	47: Try another problem. Build a word that means "an effect (usually a disease) of poison upon the skin." *toxic o derm*

toxic/o/derm

abnormally decreased
abnormally increased
combining
internal

	48: Now try a little review.
	hypo means ___*abnormally decreased*___
	hyper means ___" *increased*___
	end/o· is a ___*combining*___ form that refers to ___*internal*___ structures of the body.

	49: A little more review.
	A substance that counteracts living organisms is called an

anti/bio
external

Somat/o

___*anti bio*/tic.___

Ect/o refers to ___*external*___ structures or tissues of the body.

___*Somat o*___ / metr / y ___ means "measurement of the entire body."

By now you should have a pretty good understanding of the system of health sciences professional terminology, and you should have learned a few words and word parts as well.

REVIEW LIST

The list of words learned in this unit is for your personal use. The number beside each word indicates the question in which you learned that word or word part. Space is provided for you to make notes for review.

input (1)	ect/o (24)
practice (2)	derm (25)
feedback (4)	-gen/ic (28)
root (10)	bio- (29)
hypo- (13)	anti- (31)
hyper- (14)	febrile (35)
emia (16)	somat/o (38)
combining form (18)	ser/o (42)
fibr/o (19)	toxic/o, toxin (44)
end/o (23)	

New information - Input -
2. Practice - New information,
1. - Feedback - Correcting practice
0. - Root - Word base ..
3. - Hyper - Abnormally decreased
4. - Hyper - " increased
16 - emia - Condition of the blood
18 - Combining form - Adding a vowel

UNIT 2

Directions: Now that you have practiced using the self-instructional method in Unit 1, you are ready to begin building your health science vocabulary. Work with this unit just as you did with Unit 1. Cover the answers in the left-hand margin with your cover card. As you fill in each blank, slide the card down to check your answer.

Here's a quick review:

1: In the word *micr/o/scop/ic*,

roots
    micr and scop are ___*roots*___

combining form
    micr/o is the ___*combining form*___

ending
    ic is the ___*ending*___

(Did you remember them all? If not, try again.)

2: In the word *acr/o/megal/y*,

ending
    y is the ___*ending*___

combining form
    acr/o is the ___*combining form*___

root
    megal is a ___*root*___

3: *Cephal/o* appears in words that refer to the head. Whenever you see the combining form cephal/o in any

head
    word, you should think of the ___*root*___ .

4: Wherever the forms *cephal* or *cephal/o* appear in a word,

head
    they mean "head." The word *cephal/ic* refers to the ___*head*___

5: To build a word that refers to the head, you use the

cephal/o
    combining form ___*cephalo*___ or the root

cephal
___*cephal*___

6: In the term *en/cephal/itis*, the root cephal refers to the

head
___*head*___ .

7: The word root *alg* means "pain." Health science terms

pain
    containing alg refer to ___*pain*___ .

8: The word root *alg* means "pain." The *suffix* form (ending form) *alg/ia* refers to a body part that is experiencing

pain
___*pain*___ .

13

alg	9: To build words that refer to the sensation of pain, you use the word root _alg_
pain	10: *Cephal/alg/ia* means "a sensation of _pain_ in the head."
cephal/alg/ia	11: The word *headache* is a layman's word for the clinical term _Cephal alg / ia_ .
alg/ia	12: A general dental term meaning "toothache" is dent/ / .
	13: In the study of pharmacy or pharmacology, you must know which drugs relieve pain. Pain-relieving drugs are called *analgesics*. You know that the word "analgesic" refers
alg	to pain because you recognize the word part _alg_ .
	14: The prefix *en-* means "inside of" or "to put into or onto." Adding en-, to cephal, we build a word that refers to the
inside	_inside_ of the head.
	15: Whenever you see the word parts *en/cephal* or *en/cephal/o*,
inside	you should think of the _inside_ of the head.
	16: Since the brain is the most important organ located inside
brain	the head, the term *en/cephal* often refers to the _head brain_ .
	17: To build words referring to the brain, you should use the
en/cephal	form _en / cephal_ .
	18: The term *en/cephal/itis* refers to an inflamed condition of
brain	the covering of the _brain_ .
	19: The suffix *-oma* means "tumor." Whenever you see the
tumor	suffix -oma, you should think of a _tumor_ .
	20: A *fibroma* is a specific kind of tumor. You know the
oma	words refers to tumor when you see the suffix _oma_ .
	21: To build words that refer to tumor, you use the suffix
oma	_oma_ .
	22: The term that means "a tumor of the brain" is
oma	en/ cephal / _oma_ .
	23: Build a word that means "a tumor of the head."
cephal/oma	_Cephal / oma_
	24: The suffix *-oid* means "having a similarity to" an organ or a condition. To form a word meaning "having a similarity
oid	to the brain," you use the suffix _oid_ .
	25: Build a word meaning "having a similarity to the brain" or
en/cephal/oid	"brain-like." _en / cephal / oid_
	26: Since the word element *dent* refers to teeth, a toothlike
oid	formation would be called dent/ _oid_ .

dentalgia	27: Here's a review. The clinical term for toothache is *dentalgia*
	28: *Derm, derma,* and *dermat/o* are all word elements that refer to the skin. To build words referring to the skin, you
derm, derma, dermat/o	will most often use *derm*, *derma*, or *dermat/o*.
	29: Sometimes the root *derm* is substituted for *dermat.* Anytime you see a word containing derm or dermat, you
skin	should think of *skin*.
	30: Build a word that means "a sensation of pain in the skin."
dermat	*derm*/alg/ia
	31: A word that means "an inflammation of the skin" is
dermat	*dermalg*/itis.
	32: *Cyan* is a word root that means "blue in color." The combining form that means "blue in color" is
cyan/o	~~*dermatocyan*~~ *cyan/o*
	33: A blue color in the skin is usually caused by an insufficiency of oxygen-bearing blood reaching the skin. A child who has been swimming too long in cold water may exhibit a blue color in the skin, a condition called
cyan/o	*Cyan/o*/derm/a.
	34: Build a word that means "a sensation of pain in the skin."
dermat/alg/ia	*dermat alg i a*
	35: Build a word that means "an inflammation of the skin."
dermat/itis	*dermat itis*
	36: Anytime you see the suffix *itis*, you should think of
inflammation	*inflemation*.
inflammation	37: Encephalitis is an *inflemation* of the brain or brain covering.
	38: *Gnath/o* is the combining form that refers to the lower jaw. Any word containing gnath or gnath/o refers to the
lower jaw	*jaw*.
	39: A word that describes a condition of the lower jaw will
gnath or gnath/o	contain the word part *gnath*.
	40: In the terms *gnathology, gnathoplasty,* and *gnathoschisis,*
gnath/o	the word part that refers to the lower jaw is *gnath o*.
	41: Build a word that means "an inflammation of the lower
gnath/itis	jaw." *gnath itis*
	42: Build a word that means "pain in the lower jaw."
gnath/alg/ia	~~*alg iat gnatha*~~ *gnath alg ia*

osis

43: The suffix *-osis* usually means "an abnormal condition of a body part." A health science term referring to a diseased body part may often end with the suffix ___*osis*___ .

cyan/osis

44: The suffix *-osis* means "an abnormal condition." An abnormal bluish coloring may be called cyan/ *osis* .

osis

45: A *tubercule* is a hard, raised area on tissue or bone. An abnormal condition characterized by the presence of such raised areas is called tubercul/ *osis* .

dermat/osis

46: Build a word that means "an abnormal condition of the skin." *dermatosis*

osis

47: The term *scler* is a combining form meaning hard. (Note the absence of an "o" in this combining form.) A term meaning "an abnormal condition of hardening" is scler/ *osis* .

(The remaining questions will give you a chance to review some of what you have learned in this unit.)

cephal
en
itis
inflammation of the
  brain or brain covering

48: In the word *encephalitis*,
___*cephal*___ means "head"
___*en*___ means "inside"
___*itis*___ means "inflammation"
The word *encephalitis* means ___*inflamation*___.
___*of the brain*___

alg

49: To build words that refer to pain, you use the word root ___*alg*___ .

dentalgia

50: A word that means "toothache" is ___*dentalgia*___.

gnath/alg/ia

51: Supply the parts for the word meaning "pain of the lower jaw." *gnath algia*

dermatosis

52: A word that means "an abnormal condition of the skin" is ___*dermatosis*___ .
dermatosis

REVIEW LIST

This list of words is for your personal use. The number beside each word indicates the question in Unit 2 in which you began learning that word or word part. Space is provided for you to make notes for review.

cephal/o (3)

alg, alg/ia (7)

en- (14)

encephal (16)

-oma (19)

-oid (24)

dent (26)

derm, derma, dermat/o (28)

-itis (31)

cyan, cyan/o (32)

gnath, gnath/o (38)

-osis (43)

cephala — head

alg algia — pain

en — inside

encephal — inside head

oma — tumor / similar

oid ↗

dent — tooth

derm — derma — dermato — skin

itis — inflmation

cyan — cyano — bluish color

gnath — gnatho — lower jaw

osis — abnormal condition

Review Test for Units 1 & 2

Directions: This review test is designed to help you check your learning progress. It covers the material presented in Units 1 and 2. *This is NOT a test to be graded.* It is for your use only. You will not need to use your cover card with this review test. You should work through the test completely, trying to fill in all the blanks. Only when you have honestly tried to answer every question in this test should you turn to the answers on page 20.

1: Identify the parts of the following terms:

a) **acrodermatitis**

first combining form _derma_

ending _itis_

second root _litis_

word element meaning "inflammation" _itis_

word element meaning "skin" _derma_

b) **encephalalgia**

prefix _en_

word element meaning "pain" _alg_

ending _ia_

word element meaning "head" _cephal_

meaning of the word "encephalalgia" _Pain inside the head_

c) **cyanoderma**

combining form meaning "blue in color" _cyan_

word element meaning "skin" _derma_

19

2:   Build a word that means "pain in the lower jaw." *en 1cyano1algia*

3:   Build a word that means "causing or giving rise to poisons." *toxid o1gaiic*

4:   When you add a vowel to a root, you create a word form called a *Combing form*

5:   Build a word that means "an abnormal condition of the skin." *Derma1tosis*

6:   Build a word that means "a tumor on the brain." *en 1cophal oma*

7:   Build a word that means "a tumorous growth of skin tissue." *Hermatoma*

8:   Build a word that means "toothlike." *dent 1 aid*

You have completed the review test for Units 1 and 2. Go over your work until you are satisfied that you have done your best. Then check your answers with the answers below. If you have any incorrect answers on this test, correct them at once. But leave a mark by those items which you missed, so that you may refer to them again in the future.

ANSWERS: UNITS 1 & 2

1.	(a)	(b)	(c)
	acr/o	en	cyan/o
	itis	alg	derm
	dermat	ia	
	itis	cephal	
	dermat	pain inside the head	

2.   gnath/alg/ia

3.   toxic/o/gen/ic

4.   combining form

5.   dermat/osis

6.   en/cephal/oma

7.   dermat/oma

8.   dent/oid

UNIT 3

Directions: This unit is designed just like Units 1 and 2. Use your cover card in the left-hand margin, sliding it down to check your answer as you fill in each blank. You're learning a lot of useful health sciences terminology, so keep working!

toward

1: The prefixes *ab-* and *ad-* appear in many health science terms. The prefix ad- means "toward," so anytime you see the prefix ad—, you should think of *toward*.

ad

2: Since the prefix *ad-* means "toward," you can build words that mean "toward" by using the prefix *ad*

ad; toward

3: In the words *ad/junction*, *ad/diction*, and *ad/hesion*, the prefix *ad* means *toward*.

toward

4: The root word *duct* means "a movement" or "a channel for movement." By adding the prefix ad- to duct, you build a word meaning "a movement *toward*."

movement toward

5: When a health professional uses the word *adduction*, he is probably describing a limb's *movement toward* the center of the body.

adduction

6: The movement of a limb toward the center of the body may be called *adduction*.

away from

7: The prefix *ab-* means "away from." You won't confuse ab- with ad- if you remember that ad- means "toward" and ab- means *away from*.

ab

8: You have already learned that duct means "movement" or "a channel for movement." You know that the word *ab/duction* means "a movement away from the center line of the body" when you see the prefix *ab*.

ab; away from

9: In the words *ab/sence*, *ab/errant*, and *ab/duction*, the prefix *ab* means *toward*.

abduction

10: A muscle that moves a limb away from the center line of the body performs *abduction*.

21

absorb

11: Here's a simple problem. The root *sorb* means "drawing" or "sucking," so the word that means "drawing or sucking away from" is _____*absorb*_____ .

absorption

12: The ingredients of a pharmaceutical compound pass out of the stomach and into the blood stream by the process of _____*absorption*_____ . (Think!)

13: The blood carries many individual cells. The word element *cyt/o* means "cell." In building words that refer to cells, you will use the word element _____*cyt / o*_____ .

cyt/o

14: The bloodstream carries both white and red cells. The word element *leuk/o* means "white," so *leuk/o/cytes* are white _____*cells*_____ .

cells

15: *Lymph/o/cytes* are white blood cells produced in lymphoid tissues in the body. In other words, lymphocytes are one type of _____*leuk o / cyte*_____ .

leuk/o/cyte

16: In the words *lymph/o/cyte*, *leuk/o/cyte*, and *cyt/o/plasm*, the word element _____*cyt*_____ refers to cells.

cyt

17: Here's a more complex term for you. *Leuk/o/cyt/o/pen/ia* means "an insufficiency or decrease in white blood cells."

white
cell
pen/ia

leuk/o means _____*white*_____
cyt/o means _____*cell*_____
_____*pen / ia*_____ means insufficiency or decrease.

18: If a medical technician, performing a white blood cell count, discovers an insufficiency in the white cells, he would report that the blood sample showed _____*leuk/o/cyt/o/pen/ia*_____ .

leuk/o/cyt/o/pen/ia

19: The bloodstream also carries red cells, which are called *erythrocytes*. The combining form *erythr/o* means _____*red*_____

red

20: In discussing a patient whose lab report indicated deficiencies of both red and white blood cells, you might use the terms _____*erythr/o/cyt/o/pen/ia*_____ and _____*leuk/o/cyt/o/pen/ia*_____

erythr/o/cyt/o/pen/ia
leuk/o/cyt/o/pen/ia

21: You have been using the terms *leukocyte*, *erythrocyte*, and *lymphocyte*. Because they contain the word element *cyt*, all these terms refer to types of _____*cells*_____ .

cells

22: From word parts that you have learned build a new term for "abnormally white skin." (Think!) _____*leuk/o/derma*_____

leuk/o/derma

23: Speaking of skin, you might be interested to know that *tom/e* is a word element that means "a cutting instrument." In fact, the word element *tom* refers to cutting wherever it appears. Even if you don't know the meaning

tom	of the entire term *hepat/o/tom/y*, you recognize ___*tom*___ as referring to cutting.
	24: The term *gastr/ectomy* means "an excision (removal) of all or part of the stomach." *Gastr/o* refers to the stomach,
excision or removal	so the suffix *-ectomy* means ___*removal.*___
	25: The *duodenum* is that portion of the intestine just below the stomach (the combining form is duoden/o), so an
ectomy	excision of all or part of the duodenum is a duoden/___*ectomy*___
	26: An excision of both the stomach and the duodenum is a
duoden	gastr/o/ ___*duoden*___ ectomy.
	27: A removal of all or part of the duodenum is a *duoden-ectomy*. But an operation that merely cuts into the duodenum is a duoden/*otomy*. When a surgeon cuts into
o/tomy	the duodenum, he performs a duoden/ ___*otomy*___
	28: When a surgeon cuts into the stomach, he performs a
gastr/o/tomy	___*Gastr O Tomy*___ . (Think!)
	29: The combining form *crani/o* refers to the skull. Surgery
crani/o/tomy	that involves cutting into the skull is a ___*crani O Tomy*___
	30: You are now able to build a word that means "inflamma-
gastr/itis	tion of the stomach." ___*Gastritis*___
	31: An organ that looks like or functions like the stomach
gastr/oid	would be described as ___*Gastroid*___
	32: A condition that affects both the stomach and the
gastr/o	intestinal tract is called ___*Gastr O*___ /intestinal.
	33: The prefix *intra-* means "within." A word that means
intra	"within the stomach" is ___*intra*___ /gastr/ic.
	34: Whenever you see the prefix *intra-*, you know that it
within	means ___*Within*___ a body part.
	35: If the suffix *-ic* is an adjective ending, build a word that
intra/cephal	means "within the head." ___*intra Cephal*___ /ic.
	36: Do not confuse *intra-* with the prefix *inter-*, which means "between." Whenever you see the prefix inter-, you
between	should think of ___*between*___
	37: If a clinical psychologist is speaking of action between
inter	two patients, he uses the term ___*inter*___ /action.
	38: Build a word that means "between the teeth."
inter/dent/al	___*inter dental*___
between	39: Always remember that *inter/digit/al* means "___*between*___
within	the fingers," whereas *intra/crani/al* means "___*within*___ the cranium."
	40: *Thorac/o* is the combining form that refers to the chest.

intra/thorac

chest

thorac/otomy
thorac/ic

thorac/o/centesis

intra/thorac/ic

infra

below

infra/duoden/al

infra/gnath/ic
below

above

supra

supra/gastr/ic

ectomy

duoden/otomy

gastr/o/centesis

Use the adjective suffix, -ic to build a word that means "within the chest." *Intra thoric*

41: Whenever you see any form of *thorac/o*, you should think of the ___*Chest*___ .

42: Surgery that involves cutting into the stomach is called a *gastrotomy*. Cutting into the chest is called *thorac otomy*

43: General pain in the chest is called _____ / _____ pain.

44: *Centesis* is a word part (usually a suffix) that means "a surgical puncture." Use the suffix -centesis to build a word that means "a surgical puncture of the chest." *thorac /o/ centesis*

45: *Hemorrhage* is a word that means "bleeding." Supply the word needed to make up a term meaning "bleeding within the chest cavity." *intrathora* hemorrhage

46: The prefix *infra-* means "below." Since the abdomen is located below the chest, one could say that it is in an *infra*/thorac/ic position.

47: *Infra-* is a prefix that always means "below." Whenever you see infra-, you should think of *below* .

48: The suffix *-al*, like the suffix -ic, makes a word an adjective. Use this suffix and the correct prefix to build a word meaning "below the duodenum." *infra/ duoden al*

49: Build an adjective that means "below the lower jaw." *infra/gnath ic*

50: Never confuse *infra-*, which means *below*, with *supra*, which means "above." Whenever you see the prefix supra-, think of *above*.

51: Whenever you are describing one body part as being above another, you should use the prefix *supra* .

52: Use the *-ic* suffix to build a word meaning "above the stomach." *supra gastric*

53: A diagnosis of cancer of the stomach may indicate excision (surgical removal) of all or part of the stomach. Such a procedure is called a gastr/*e otomy*

54: An exploration of the area of the duoden/um may require a surgical incision into the duodenum. Such a procedure is called a *duoden otomy*

55: The surgical puncture of the stomach is called a *Gastr o/ centesis*

ostomy

56: The suffix *-ostomy* describes a surgical procedure. When a new opening is created in a body part, such as the stomach, that operation is described by using the suffix -ostomy. To describe the surgical creation of a new opening, use the suffix _ostomy_

opening

57: Surgery to create a more or less permanent new opening in a body part is described by the suffix *-ostomy*. When you see -ostomy, you should think of a new _opening_

ostomy

58: When it becomes necessary to make a new opening in the stomach, a gastr/_ostomy_ is performed.

duoden/ostomy

59: Build a word that means "the creation of a new opening in the duodenum." _duodenostomy_

duoden/ostomy

60: The dysfunction of the natural opening between the stomach and the duodenum (the infragastric portion of the small intestine) may require the creation of a new opening between them. Such surgery is called a gastr/o_duodenostomy_

(Note how the parts of the word you just built fit together, using one combining form but not the other.)

otomy
ostomy
ectomy

61: Complete this question and discover a way to remember the distinctions among the three main surgical suffixes.
making a surgical incision _otomy_
making a more permanent opening _ostomy_
cutting out a body tissue _ectomy_

adduction

62: The movement of a limb toward the center of the body is called _adduction_

white blood cells

63: *Leukocytopenia* means "an insufficiency or decrease in _white blood cells_

within the stomach
between the teeth

64: The word *intragastric* means _within the stomach_ the word *interdental* means _between the teeth_

supra/gnath/ic

65: Build a word that means "above the lower jaw." _supragnathic_

duoden/itis

66: Build a word that means "an inflammation of the duodenum." _duodenitis_
Build a word that means "an abnormal condition of the

gastr/osis

stomach." _gastrosis_

You have completed Unit 3. Look over your work carefully. You may work through the entire unit again, if you would like to.

REVIEW LIST

This list of words is for your personal use. The number beside each word indicates the question in Unit 3 in which you began learning that word or word part. Space is provided for you to make notes for review.

ad- (1) *toward*

adduction (4) *toward*

ab- (7) *away from*

abduction (10) *away from centerline*

absorption (11) *absorb*

cyt/o (13) *cell*

leukocyte (15) *white blood cell*

-penia (17) *decrease*

erythr/o (19) *red cells*

tom (23) *cutting*

-ectomy (24) *removal*

gastr/o, duoden/o (26) *stomach & duoden...*

-otomy (27) *incision into*

crani/o (29) *skull*

intra- (33) *within*

inter- (36) *between*

thorac/o (40) *chest*

centesis (44) *surgical puncture*

infra- (46) *below*

supra- (50) *above*

-ostomy (56) *surgical opening*

UNIT 4

Directions: Please use your cover card in working through this unit just as you did in the three previous units. Remember, if you have difficulty with any instructions or are unsure about any of the content of this unit, ask your instructor.

Quick Review:

gastrotomy

1: A surgical incision into the stomach is called a
   gastrotomy

A surgical removal of part or all of the lower jaw is called a

gnathectomy

   gnathectomy

Surgery that makes a new opening between the stomach

gastroduodenostomy

   and the duodenum is called a *gastroduodentomy*
   A condition that exists within the head may be described

intracephal

   as *intracephalic*

2: The word *sepsis* means "infection." It is a noun. When
   you, as a health professional, need to refer to a condition

sepsis

   of infection, you will use the word _*sepsis*_ .

3: Call upon your memory for a word element that you
   learned in an earlier unit. Build a term that means "coun-

anti/sepsis

   teracting infection *anti/sepsis*

4: The prevention of the growth of infection-causing micro-

anti/sepsis

   organisms is called *anti/sepsis*

5: You have already built words in which the suffix *-ic*
   makes the word an adjective. Now use -ic to build a word
   (an adjective) that describes a drug or other chemical com-

anti/sep/tic

   pound that fights infection *anti/sep/tic*

(Did that change of letter throw you? It's like the letter
change that you learned in bio/tic. Remember it!)

6: You've already learned that the suffix *-al* may also be used
   to make a word an adjective. Use -al to build a word that

27

anti/malari

means "preventing disease caused by the malaria parasite." *Anti Malari al*

7: The suffix -*ant* may make a word either an adjective or a noun. Use -ant to build a term that means "preventing the coagulation of blood." (Think!) *Anti Coagul ant*

anti/coagul/ant

8: In building the word in Question 7, you discovered the root that refers to the change of a liquid into a jellylike state. What is that root? *Coagul*

coagul

9: A drug that is administered to stop bleeding by changing the blood from a liquid into a jellylike state is a *Coagul ant*

coagul/ant

10: In contrast to the word that you built in Question 9, build a word that describes a drug administered to make blood thinner, or less likely to coagulate. *anti coagul ant*

anti/coagul/ant

11: The prefixes *a-* and *an-* are two different forms of the same prefix. Both mean "not" or "without," but a- is used before a consonant (a/sepsis) and an- is used before a vowel (an/esthesia). Whenever you see the prefixes a- or an-, you should think of *not* or *Without*

not, without

12: To build a word that means "not" or "without," you should use the prefix *an* before a vowel and the prefix *a* before a consonant.

an, a

13: Now try putting that piece of information to work.
a/sepsis means "without infection"
a derm ic means "without skin"
an /enter/ous means "without an intestine"
a /gastr/ ic means "without a stomach"
an /ox/ia means "without normal oxygen"

a/sepsis
a/derm
an
a/gastr
an

(If you made all or most of the right choices in Question 13, you are to be congratulated. So, congratulations!)

14: Now choose the correct endings to build words that mean "a drug that fights infection": *anti septic*
"without malaria" *a malari al*
"without infection" (adjective) *a sep tic*

anti/sep/tic
a/malari/al
a/sep/tic

15: The term *antagonist* refers to any drug, muscle, and so on, that tends to resist or fight against another. The part of this term that means "against is _____ .

an

16: The word *leukemia* is sometimes said to mean "white blood." Look closely at the word parts that make up the an/em/ia

word leukemia, then build a word which means (literally, but not clinically) "without blood." *anemia*

17: Use the correct suffix to build a word that describes the condition of insufficient red blood cells (without blood). *anemic*

an/em/ic

18: Here are three health science terms that look very much alike: *anabolism*, *catabolism*, and *metabolism*. The word part *-bolism* in each tells you that the word refers to the basic chemical processes of living organisms. A quick glance at each word tells you that they refer to the basic chemical processes of living organisms because you see the word part *bolism*

bolism

the basic chemical
  processes of living
  organisms

19: In each word in Question 18, the word part *-bolism* refers to *the basic chemical processes of living organisms*

20: The prefix ana- in *ana/bolism* tells you that simple chemical substances are synthesizing (joining together) to create complex substances. The prefix that specifies the synthesizing of chemical substances is *ana*

ana

21: When nutritive matter is synthesized into living substance, the process is called *anabolism*

ana/bolism

22: The prefix *cata-* means the opposite of ana-. When the complex substances break down into simple substances, the process is called *cata*bolism.

cata

23: In the words *cata/bolic* and *cata/tonic*, the word part meaning "breaking down from complex to simple" is *cata*

cata

24: In the words *ana/bolism* and *cata/bolism*, the prefix ana- means *synthesizing*, the prefix cata- means *breaking down*.

synthesizing,
  breaking down

25: The third word, *metabolism*, also refers to a chemical process of a living organism. The word part that refers to the chemical process of a living organism is *bolism*

bolism

26: The prefix *meta-* means "change." When you see such words as meta/phase and meta/bolism, you know some change is described by the word part *meta*

meta

27: The term *meta/bolism* has a larger meaning than either anabolism or catabolism. Metabolism refers to the *total* chemical process of a living organism. The process that includes both anabolism (synthesizing) and catabolism (breaking down) is *Metal aolism*

meta/bolism

28: Both anabolism and catabolism are essential processes in producing and sustaining the living organism. The word that means "the total of the chemical processes of a living organism" is *metabolism*

metabolism

29: The processes that include both the change of nutrients to living substance and the breaking down of living substance are summed up in the word *metabolism*

metabolism

30: When substances in the body are broken down and converted into energy, the process of *catabolism* is taking place.

catabolism

31: Infants are occasionally born with a defect called *macro-cephalism* in which the head is extremely large and some degree of retardation is usually exhibited. Look carefully at the word macro/cephalism, meaning "large head." Which part of the word means "large"? *macro*

macro

32: Using the -ic adjective suffix, build a word that means "having an abnormally large head." *macro cephal ic*

macro/cephal/ic

33: Build a word that means "an abnormally large red blood cell." *Macro erythro cyte*

macro/erythr/o/cyte

34: The combining form *odont/o* refers to tooth or the teeth. Build a word that means "an abnormally large tooth" or "abnormally large teeth." *Macro dont*ism.

macro/dont

(Did the letter change trip you up? In building health sciences terms, you will rarely use a double vowel such as "oo" between word parts.)

35: Remember that the suffix -ia means "a condition of the body or a body part." Can you build a word that means "a condition of abnormal stomach enlargement"? Try it. *macro gastr ia*

macro/gastr/ia

36: The prefix *micro*- means the opposite of macro-. So if an infant is born with an abnormally small head, his condition is called. *Micro*cephal/ism.

micro

37: A laboratory instrument designed for examining very small objects is called a *micro*scope.

micro

38: The word part *meter* means "an instrument for measuring." An instrument designed to measure in very small units is a *Micro*meter.

micro

39: The word part *ambul* appears in several health sciences terms. It refers to moving from place to place. In words such as ambul/ant, ambul/ance, and ambul/atory, the act of moving from place to place is specified by the word

ambul

part *ambul*.

ambul

40: An *ambul/ance* is a vehicle for moving sick or injured persons from place to place. A patient whose disease does not confine him to bed is called an *ambul*atory patient.

ambul

41: A patient who is hospitalized with a dermatosis may still be able to walk from place to place. This patient is able to *ambul*/ate.

ambulatory

42: An automobile accident victim who, although injured, can still walk is described as being *ambulatory*

43: The word part *lip* (combining form lip/o) refers to "fat." Consequently, a word that means "accumulation of fat in

lip

the tissues" is *lip* /o/pexia.

lip/o

44: When the heart muscle begins to degenerate into fatty tissue, the condition is called *lip* /o/cardia.

45: Think back to a word element that you learned in an earlier unit, an element meaning "giving rise to" or "causing." Then build a term that means "giving rise to or

lip/o/gen/ic

causing fat or fatness." *lipogenic*

46: Try building a few more words which use elements that you have already learned:

lip/o/cyte   *lipocyte* means "a fat cell"
lip/ectomy   *lipectomy* means "excision of fatty tissue"
lip/o   *lip/o*/pen/ia means "a reduction of fats in the blood"

47: Another common word element in health science terminology is *iso-*, which means "equal." The term that describes equality of size in the pupils of the eyes is

iso

iso /coria.

48: In a certain kind of exercise, the muscle fibers do not change in measure or length. This is popularly called

iso

iso /metric exercise.

49: A lens that transmits light equally in all directions is called

iso

an *iso* /tropic lens.

50: A radiation therapist may prescribe a radiation dose (the key word is *dose*) of the same number of roentgens. Such

iso/dose

a dose is an *iso* /dose

51: When an infant is born with a larger than normal head, the

macro/cephal

condition is referred to as *macro cephal*ism.

meta/bolism

anti/septic

lip/o/cata

a

52: The total of all chemical processes in a living organism is called *meta bolism*

53: A medicinal agent used against infection is an *anti septic*

54: The process by which complex fatty substances are broken down into simpler substances would be called *lip/o/cata*/bolism. Think!

55: An organism that has no stomach would be described as *a*/gastr/ic.

You have completed Unit 4. Review your work carefully.

REVIEW LIST

This list of words learned in this unit is for your personal use. The number beside each word indicates the question in which you learned that word or word part. Space is provided for you to make notes for review.

sepsis (2) *infection*

coagul (7) *Coagulation of blood*

a-, an- (11) *not or without*

anemia (16) *without blood*

anabolism (20) *joining together*

catabolism (22) *breaking down (simpler substance)*

metabolism (26) *Changed*

macro- (31) *large*

micro- (36) *small*

ambul (39) *moveable*

lip/o (43) *refers to fat*

iso- (47) *equal*

Review Test for Units 3 & 4

Directions: This review test is designed to help you check your learning progress. It covers the material presented in Units 3 and 4. *This is NOT a test to be graded.* It is for your use only. You will not need to use your cover card with this review test. You should work through the test completely, trying to fill in all the blanks. Only when you have honestly tried to answer every question in this test should you turn to the answers on page 34.

1: Remembering the prefixes ad- and ab-, build a word that describes the action of a muscle moving a limb toward the center of the body. *ab /duction*

2: Use the word elements listed below to build the correct health science terms called for:

cyt/o	leuk/o	erythr/o
pen/ia	duoden/o	otomy
ectomy	crani/o	ostomy

   a) word that means "an incision into the skull" *Craniotomy*

   b) word that means "a decrease in red blood cells" *erythrocytopenia / leukocytopenia*

   c) word that means "white blood cell" *cyto leukocyte*

   d) word that means "excision of part or all of the duodenum" *duodenotomy*

3: Bleeding that occurs within the chest cavity can be called *intrathoracic* hemorrhage.

4: If you wished to locate a diseased body part above the stomach, you could describe it as *supragastric* .

5: Use the suffix -al in building a word to describe an intestinal area below the duodenum. *infraduodenal*

6: The word that may describe the way an anesthetic gas enters the bloodstream from the lungs literally means "sucking away from." What is that word? *absorption*

7: Use the -ant ending to build a word which describes any factor that prevents blood from changing into a jellylike state. *anticoagulant*

8: What word (a noun) means "an infection-free condition"? *asepis*

9: Think of the basic chemical processes of living organisms. When nutritive matter is synthesized into living substance, the process is called *anabolism*. When substances in the body are broken down and converted into energy, the process is called *Catabolism*. The two processes you have just named are summed up in the single term *metabolism*.

10: Words that name or describe things of equal characteristics often use the word element *iso*.

11: An infant born with an abnormally large head is described as *Macrocephalic*. (Use the correct adjective ending.)

12: The combining form lip/o generally refers in some way to *fat*.

13: In your notebook rewrite the following sentence in nonprofessional, or layman's, terms.

The patient complained of supragastric pain. An exploratory thoracotomy was performed. Evidence of intrathoracic sepsis was found, as well as indications of lipocardia.

You have completed the review test for Units 3 and 4. Go over your work until you are satisfied that you have done your best. Then check your answers with the answers below. If you have any incorrect answers on this test, correct them at once. But leave a mark by those items which you missed, so that you may refer to them again in the future.

ANSWERS: UNITS 3 & 4

1. ad/duction

2. (a) craniotomy; (b) erythrocytopenia; (c) leukocyte; (d) duodenectomy

3. intrathoracic

4. supragastric

5. infraduodenal

6. absorption

7. anticoagulant

8. asepsis

9. anabolism; catabolism; metabolism

10. iso

11. macrocephalic

12. fat

13. The patient complained of pain located above the stomach. An exploratory incision into the chest was performed. Evidence of infection within the chest was found, as well as indications of the heart muscle degenerating into fatty tissue.

UNIT 5

Directions: Proceed as in the previous units. Be sure to use your cover card.

1: Again, we begin with a short review. A word meaning "the synthesizing of simple substances into complex ones": *anabolism* A word meaning "a condition of abnormally large teeth": *macrodontism* A word describing a radiation dose of the same number of roentgens: *isodose*

anabolism
macrodontism

isodose

2: The word element *alveo* means "a hollow cavity." Whenever you see the word element alveo, you should think of a *hollow cavity*

hollow cavity

3: The word element *alveo* appears in words referring to the sockets of the teeth (dental alveoli) or to the thin-walled chambers of the lungs (pulmonary alveoli). Whenever you use a word that refers to one of these hollow cavities, you will probably use a form of the word element *alveo*.

alveo

4: The term *alveolalgia* means "pain in the socket of an extracted tooth." The part of the word that means pain is *algia*. The part of the word that refers to the tooth socket is *alveo*.

algia
alveo
inflammation of a
  tooth socket

5: What is the dental science meaning of the term *alveolitis*? *inflammation of a tooth socket*

6: The prefix *para-* has several distinct meanings. It may mean "abnormal," as in para/functional (not functioning normally). It may also mean "involving two parts," as in para/site (an organism drawing nourishment from another). The prefix *para* may appear in words meaning either "abnormal" or "involving two parts."

para

7: *Paralalia* is a term meaning "a defect or abnormality of speech." Which part of the term refers to abnormality? *para*

para

37

para

para/   /ectomy

para/pineal/ectomy

para/noia

para

para/neur

neur/o

neur/itis
neur/algia
neur/o/cyte

neur/al

neurectomy

neur/o/gastr/ic

neur/o/muscul

neuromuscular

8: The prefix *para-* may also mean "beside" or "near." This is the usage in the word *para/thyroid*, which refers to glands that are adjacent to the thyroid gland. The word part *cystic* refers to the bladder, so the tissue near the bladder is described as *para/*cystic.

9: The excision, or surgical removal, of the parathyroid glands is called a *para/*thyroid/ *ectomy*

10: The excision of tissue adjacent to the pineal is called a *para/pineal/ectomy*

11: Don't forget the other meanings of para-. If the word element *noia* means "to think," what word means "to think abnormally"? *para noia*

12: When studying community health needs, public health researchers often use a paradigm, or model, of the community. The part of the term which tells you that the model is similar ("near") to the real community is *para*

13: The combining form *neur/o* refers to a nerve. Tissue that is adjacent to nerve tissue is called *para neur/*al   tissue.

14: *Neur/o* refers to a nerve, so you should think of a nerve or the nervous system whenever you see the combining form *neur/o*.

15: Build a word that means "inflammation of nerve tissue." *neur/itis*

16: Pain in the nerve tissue is *neur/al/gia*

17: A nerve cell of any kind is called a *neur/o/cyte*

18: The adjective suffix *-al* means "relating to." Use this suffix to build a word meaning "relating to any part of the nervous system." *neur/al*

19: It is sometimes necessary to excise, or remove, a segment of a nerve. This surgical procedure is called a *neurectomy*

20: Build a compound word that refers to the nerves of the stomach. *neur/o/gastr/ic*

21: The combining form *muscul/o* appears in words referring to a muscle or the muscular system. A word that refers to the nerve supply of a muscle is *neur/o/muscul/ar*

22: The word that you built in Question 21 is also used to refer jointly to nerves and muscles. A word meaning "relating to both nerves and muscles" is *neuromuscular*

23: Forms of the Greek word *logos* appear in many health

science terms. Logos means "knowledge" or "study."
(Think of the word "logic.") The suffix that means "the
study of" is *-logy*. Build a word that means "the study of

neur/o/logy   the nervous system." *neurology*

24: The suffix *-ist* usually means "one who." Now build a
word meaning "one who studies the stomach."

gastr/o/log/ist   *gastrologist*

25: The *-al* suffix is used to build adjectives that refer to the
study of a body part or function. Use this suffix to build a
word that refers to the study of the nervous system.

neur/o/logic/al   *neurological*

26: The combining form *path/o* means "disease" or "abnormal condition." Whenever you see any form of *path/o*

path/o   you should think of disease or abnormal condition.

27: The study of disease—its nature, causes, and develop-
path/o/logy   ment—is called *pathology*

28: The study of disease of the tissues of the oral cavity is
pathology   called dental *pathology*.

29: A two-word term that means "the study of diseases or
neuromuscular   abnormalities of the body's nervous and muscular sys-
   pathology   tems" is *neuromuscular pathology*

30: A single compound word that means "one who studies
diseases or abnormalities of the nervous system" is

neuropathologist   *neuropathologist*

31: The combining form *eti/o* comes from a Greek word
meaning "cause." Use this combining form to build a
word meaning "the study of the causes of disease."

eti/o/logy   *etiology*

32: Use the *-al* suffix to build a word that refers to the study
eti/o/logic/al   of the causes of disease. *etiological*

33: If you wished to refer to a specific condition which was
the cause of a specific disease, you would describe that
condition as etiopathic. The part of this word that means

etio   "cause" is *etio* The part that means "disease" is
pathic   *pathic*

34: If a laboratory analysis indicates that a certain organism
has caused a disease, that organism could be described as

etiopathic   *etiopathic*

35: The prefix *dia-* means "throughout" or "completely."

When it is combined with the word part *gnosis*, the meaning is "to know completely." When a physician determines what disease is causing a patient's symptoms, he knows the disease completely and has achieved a

dia/gnosis *dia gnosis*

36: The practice of determining ("knowing completely") the nature of a disease by examination of symptoms is called

dia/gnosis *dia gnosis*

37: When building words with the prefix *dia-*, you must sometimes drop the letter "a." Keep this in mind as you combine dia- with the word part uresis (urination) to build a

di/uresis word meaning "complete urination." *diuresis*

38: The word *diuresis* generally means "excessive urination." Sometimes when the body is producing and passing too

diuresis much urine, the condition is called *diuresis*.

39: In some cases, the body does not produce or pass a sufficient amount of urine. Then a medication may be prescribed to cause a normal or even abnormal amount of

di/ure urine to pass. Such a medication is called a *diuretic*.

40: If the body does not pass waste as urine at a normal rate,

diuretic a *diuretic* may be administered to increase the amount of urine passed.

41: The combining form *abdomin/o* is used in words that refer to the large body cavity containing the stomach, intestines, liver, and other organs. The combining form for

abdomin/o words referring to the area of the abdomen is *abdomin/o*

42: Pain that occurs simultaneously in the chest and in the

abdomin/o abdomen is described as *abdomin/o* thorac/ic pain.

43: Whenever you see the word root *abdomin*, you should

abdomen think of the area of the *abdomen*

44: The chest is located above the abdomen, so it could be

supra-abdomin described as *supra abdominal*

45: Bleeding that occurs within the abdominal cavity is called

intra-abdominal *intra abdomin* hemorrhage.

46: If there were a health professional who specialized in the

abdominologist study of the abdomen, he would be an *abdominologist*

47: The combining form *enter/o* refers to the intestine. Build a word that means "the study of the intestine."

enter/o/logy *enter/o/logy*

enterologist

48: One who studies the intestine is an *enterologist*

gastr/o/   /o/logist

49: A specialist (think of "one who studies") in both the stomach and the intestine is called a *gastr/o/enter/o/logist*

enterostomy

50: The surgical creation of a new opening in the intestine is called an *enterostomy*

51: Wastes produced by digestion within the intestine leave the body at the anus, which is an *orifice* or body opening. Whenever you see the word orifice, you know that it re-

opening

fers to an *opening* in the body.

52: The mouth is a natural opening in the body. The mouth

orifice

can be called an *orifice*

53: Between the stomach and the duodenum is an opening

orifice

that is called the duodenal *orifice* of the stomach.

54: Look at the word *alveolalgia.* Which word part refers to

algia

pain? *algia*

a hollow cavity

The other word part refers to *a hollow cavity*

55: The glandular tissue adjacent to the thyroid gland is called

para

the *para*thyroid gland.

56: What is the word that means (literally, but not clinically)

para

"to think abnormally"? *paranoia* Which part of this

para

word means "abnormal"? *para*

57: Build a word that refers jointly to nerves and muscle.

neur/o/muscul/ar

neural-muscular

58: What compound word means "one who studies diseases or

neuropathologist

abnormalities of the nervous system"? *neuropathologist*

59: A medication administered to increase the flow of urine is

diuretic

called a *diuretic.*

60: Finally, build a word that means "an operation to create a new opening between the stomach and the intestine."

gastr/o/enter/ostomy

gastroenterostomy

You have completed Unit 5. Look over your work carefully. You may work through the entire unit again, if you feel that you need to do so.

REVIEW LIST

This list of words is for your personal review. The number beside each word indicates the question in Unit 5 in which you began learning that word or word part. Space is provided for you to make notes for review.

alveo (2) *A hollow cavity*   **eti/o** (31) *Cause*

para- (6) *in a lack of two parts*   **dia-** (35) *Completely*

neur/o (13) *nerve*   **abdomin/o** (41) *Stomach cavity*

muscul/o (21) *muscle*   **enter/o** (47) *intestines*

-logy, -logist (23) *the study of —*   **orifice** (51) *natural opening*

path/o (26) *disease*

UNIT 6

Directions: There's nothing new in the directions for working with Unit 6. Remember that as you complete each terminology unit you are becoming better prepared for your health science student and professional career. So work hard.

1: To review, in the word *diuretic*, the prefix di(a)- means

completely, urine ___*completely*___ The word part uretic refers to ___*urine*___ .
The word *gastropathy* refers to any disease of the stom-

pathy arch. Which word part refers to disease? ___*pathy*___
orifice A natural opening into the body is called an ___*orifice*___ .

2: The combining form meaning "bone" is *oste/o.* Whenever you see or hear a word containing some form of oste/o,
bone you should think of ___*bone*___

3: *Oste/o/pathy* refers to any disease of the bone. The word
oste/o part that means "bone" is ___*oste o*___

4: Build a word that means "inflammation of bone tissue."
oste/itis ___*ostelitis*___

5: The *periosteum* is a thick membrane covering almost the entire surface of a bone. What part of the word peri-
oste osteum refers to bone? ___*oste*___

6: The prefix *peri-* means "around." The word periosteum
around means " a membrane that is ___*around*___ the bone."

7: The word periodontium means "the tissues that are around and attached to the teeth." The part of this word
odont that means "teeth" is ___*odont*___ The part of this word that
peri means "around" is ___*peri*___

8: What word means "an inflammation of the tissue around
periodontitis the teeth"? ___*periodontitis*___

9: The word *periphery* (which has both professional and nonprofessional meanings) generally means "around the

phery

outside." Which part of the word peri/phery means "outside"? _Phery_

10: Use the correct adjective suffix to build a word which describes anything that is around the outside. _peripheral_

peri/pher/al

11: The resistance of the walls of the capillaries (the small blood vessels located near the surface, or "around the outside," of the body) to the passage of blood is called _peripheral_ resistance.

peripheral

12: Because many capillaries are located near the surface of the body, the resistance that they offer to the passage of blood is called _peripheral resistance_.

peripheral resistance

13: Do you remember the health science term that literally means "white blood"? _leukemia_
What part of this word refers to blood? _em_

leukemia
em

14: There is a common prefix that also means "blood": *hemo-* or *hemato-*. (Notice that *em* appears in these prefixes.) In the term hemo/philia, which part of the word refers to blood? _hemo_

hemo

15: Using a form of the word part *cyt/o*, meaning "cell," build a word that means "any blood cell." _hemo/cyte_

hemo/cyte

16: The word *hemorrhage* means "heavy bleeding." What part of this word refers to blood? _hemo_

hemo

17: Severe bleeding within the stomach is called gastric _hemorrhage_.

hemorrhage
hemology, or
   (better) hematology

18: Build a word that means "the study of the blood." _hemology — hematology_

19: Do not confuse *hemo-* with the prefix *hemi-*, which refers to half. The term hemi/algia means "pain that afflicts one half the body." In this word, algia refers to _pain_ and hemi- refers to _half_.

pain
half

20: To build a word that means "a toxin (poison) which is half the normal strength," pharmacists add a prefix. What would the word be? _hemitoxin_

hemitoxin

21: The word that means "deformity of one half the lower jaw" is made up of word parts meaning half and lower jaw plus a suffix. Build the word _hemi/gnath_ia.

hemi/gnath

22: The word *genesis*—meaning "production" or "origin" —appears in many forms in health sciences terms. You may be fairly certain that whenever you see the word parts *geni* or *gen* that the reference is to production. In the word bi/o/genesis, the combining form bi/o refers to

life, production _life_____ and the suffix -genesis means _Production_

production of life The whole word means _production of life_

23: The word *hemogenic* is an adjective form referring to the production of blood cells. Define the word parts:

hemo _hemo_ is blood

gen _gen_ is production

ic _ic_ is the adjective ending

24: The word *pathogenic* means "producing disease." The

disease combining form *path/o* means _disease_.

producing The word part *gen* means _producing_.

Pathogenic is an adjective. The noun meaning "the process

path/o/genesis of disease production" is _path o genesis_

(If you built the right word in Question 24, you are doing very well.)

25: The word part *dist* often—but not always—means "apart" or "distant from." You may describe the wrist, for

distant example, as a distal extremity, because it is _distant_ from the trunk of the body.

26: In dental anatomy, the distal surface of a tooth is that surface which is farthest from the center of the dental arch, a point located between the two front teeth. (Think of your own mouth.) Whenever you think of a tooth's

center distal surface, think of the surface farthest from the _center_ of the arch.

27: If you were comparing the knee and the ankle, which

ankle would you describe as the distal joint? _ankle_

28: The word part *labi/o* refers to the lips. In the word *dist/o/labi/al*,

dist/o _dist o_ is farthest from center of dental arch

labi _labi_ is closest to the lips

al _al_ is the adjective ending

29: The angle formed where the distal and labial surfaces of a

distolabial tooth meet is called the _distolabial_ angle.

30: The opposite of distal is *proximal*. A body part that is closer or closest to the trunk or center line of the body

proximal can be described as _proximal_

31: If you were comparing the elbow and the shoulder, which

shoulder

would you describe as the proximal joint? _shoulder_

32: As you can probably guess, the term *medial* refers to the center or middle. A nerve or muscle that is in the center of a body part is said to be in a _medial_ position.

medial

33: Imagine yourself standing with your arms extended straight out from the shoulders. With reference to your neck, your elbows are in a ~~proximal~~ _distal_ position; your shoulders are in a _proxima_ position; your throat is in the _media_ position

distal
proximal
medial

34: The combining form *later/o* means "on the side" or "outside." To build words referring to the side, use the combining form _later / o_ .

later/o

35: The word *lateroabdominal* refers to areas on the sides of the abdomen. The word part that means "side" is _later/o_ .

later/o

36: The word *flexion* means "bending." The act of bending to one side is called _later/o_ flexion.

later/o

37: Any movement to the side is a _later_ /al movement.

later

38: The word *adenoid* means "resembling a gland" or "glandlike." The suffix meaning "resembling" is _oid_ . The word root for gland is _aden_ , and its combining form is _aden o-_ .

oid
aden
aden/o

39: Adenoid is an adjective meaning "resembling a gland." You may have had your adenoids (glandlike tissues) removed when you were a child. These glandlike tissues in the passage connecting the nose and throat are _aden/oid_ tissues.

aden/oid

40: A general term for pain in a gland is _aden/algia_ .

aden/algia

41: The excision or removal of a gland is called an _aden/ectomy_ .

aden/ectomy

42: The suffix *-oma* means "tumor." A tumor in or on a gland is called an _aden/oma_

aden/oma
duodenoma

43: A tumor of the duodenum is called a _duodenoma_

44: A tumor in or on the brain is an _encephaloma_ .

encephaloma

45: A mass of clotted blood outside a vein is described by a word that would literally mean "blood tumor." Can you build the word? _hemat/oma_

hemat/oma

46: The combining form that refers to cancer is *carcin/o.* Whenever you see some form of carcin/o, think of _cancer_.

cancer

47: The noun that means "the process of disease production" is pathogenesis. Build a word to mean "the process of producing cancerous tissue." *Carcinogenesis*

carcin/o/genesis

48: Now build a word that means "a cancerous tumor." *Carcinoma*

carcin/oma

49: A cancerous growth or tumor of the stomach would be described by the two-word term *Gastric Carcinoma*

gastric carcinoma

50: Build a word that means "a cancerous tumor in a gland." *adenocarcinoma*

aden/o/carcin/oma

51: Another word for tumor is *neoplasm*, which literally means "new growth." When a new growth of cells develops in or on body tissue, it may be called a *neoplasm*

neoplasm

52: Take a look at these word parts, since they appear in many health science terms.

neo is new

plas/m is growth or formation

A carcinoma is a type of new cell growth called a *neoplasm*

neoplasm

53: A thickening of an area of skin, caused by an abnormal new growth of skin tissue is a *dermatoma*

dermatoma

54: Divide the word *periosteum* into its component parts:

ost means bone

oste

peri means around

peri

eum is the suffix

um

55: Resistance to blood flow created in the capillaries (small vessels near the surface) is called *peripheral* resistance.

peripheral

56: Build the word that means "pain in half of the body." *hemialgia*

hemi/algia

57: Can you define the word *biogenic*? *producing life*

producing life

58: A body part that is closer to the center line of the body is in the *proximal* position; one that is farther, or farthest, from the center line is in the *distal* position.

proximal
distal

59: Inflammation of a gland is called *adenitis*.

adenitis

You have completed Unit 6. Look over your work carefully. You may wish to work through the entire unit again.

REVIEW LIST

This list of words is for your personal review. The number beside each word indicates the question in Unit 6 in which you began learning that word or word part. Space is provided for you to make notes for review.

oste/o (2) *bone*

peri- (6) *around*

periphery (9) *around the outside*

hemo-, hemato- (14) *blood*

hemi- (19) *half*

gen, -genic, genesis (22) *production*

dist/al, dist/o (25) *distant*

proximal (30) *closer*

medial (32) *center*

later/o, lateral (34)

aden/o (38) *gland*

-oma (42) *tumor*

carcin/o (46) *cancer*

neo/plas/m (51) *new tumor*

Review Test for
Units 5 & 6

Directions: This is another review test designed to help you check your learning progress. This review covers the words and word parts that you have learned in Units 5 and 6. *This is NOT a test to be graded.* It is for your use only. You will not need to use your cover card with this review test. You should work through the test completely, trying to fill in all blanks. Turn to the answers on page 50 only when you have tried to answer every question in this test.

1: Look closely at the two-word term alveolar hemorrhage. You have not learned this term, but you have learned many of the parts. Now define the term: _____

bleeding — (lungs) sac bleeding

2: You have learned three meanings of the prefix para-. Define para- as it is used in each of these terms:

a) **para/site:** para means _____ _two sights or two parts_

b) **para/noia:** para means _____ _abnormal behaviour_

c) **para/thyroid:** para means _near the thyroid_

3: Build a word that means "one who studies the nervous system." _neurologist_

4: Build a word that means "disease or abnormality of the intestine."
entero/path/ology

5: From the collection of word parts below, build health science terms that describe the following processes or conditions:

a) inflammation of both nerve tissue and bone _neuro osteitis_ /

b) referring to the tissue around the teeth _peri/odont_ /ic

c) affecting only one side of the body _hemi/later_/al

49

 d) the production of cancerous neoplasm _Carcinogenesis_

hemi-	peri-	later/o	carcin/o
-itis	neur/o	odont/o	oste/o
genesis			

6: A tumor in or on a gland is an ___*adenoma*___.

7: Severe bleeding within the chest cavity would be called ___*intrathoracic hemorrhage*___

8: On the line below you will see points A, B, and C. Use the correct terms to describe their positions in relation to the point of reference, which is X.

<pre>
        B   A   X   A   B
                  C
</pre>

 a) Point **A** is in the ___*proximal*___ position.

 b) Point **B** is in the ___*distal*___ position.

 c) Point **C** is at the ___*medial*___ position.

9: With the help given, build a word that means "a disease or abnormality involving the nervous system, the brain, and the spinal cord."   (myel/o = spinal cord)

___*neuro*___ ___*encephal*___ / /myel/o/ *pathy*

You have completed the review test for Units 5 and 6. Go over your work until you are satisfied that you have done your best. Then check your answers against the answers below. If you have any incorrect answers on this test, correct them at once. But leave a mark by those items which you missed, so that you may refer to them again in the future.

ANSWERS: UNITS 5 & 6

1. heavy bleeding of a hollow cavity (such as tooth socket or lung sacs)

2. a) para/site: para = involving two parts
    b) para/noia: para = abnormal
    c) para/thyroid: para = beside, near, or adjacent to

3. neur/o/log/ist

4. enter/o/path/y

5. (a) neur/o/oste/itis; (b) peri/odont/ic; (c) hemi/later/al; (d) carcin/o/genesis

6. adenoma

7. intrathoracic hemorrhage

8. (a) proximal; (b) distal; (c) medial;

9. neur/o/encephal/o/myel/o/path/y (neuroencelphalomyelopathy)

UNIT 7

Directions: When working with Unit 7, again keep the left-hand margin covered with your cover card. You may want to check your progress—and get some useful health sciences terminology practice—by reading in professional books and journals from time to time. If you are now in health professional school, you will find such reading particularly useful.

cardi/o

1: The combining form that refers to the heart is *cardi/o*. You know that the term *electr/o/cardi/o/gram* refers to a measurement of the electrical activity of the heart when you see the combining form *Cardio*.

heart

2: A *cardi/o/log/ist* specializes in the study and treatment of diseases of the heart. Whenever you see any form of cardi/o, you should think of the *heart*.

cardi/otomy

3: Build a word that means "a surgical incision of the heart." *Cardiotomy*

cardi

4: Build a word that means "pertaining to the heart" (and note the special adjective suffix form). *Cardi*ac

vas/o
vascul/o

5: The combining forms *vas/o* and *vascul/o* are used in words that refer to the blood vessels. You should think of blood vessels whenever you see the form *vas/o* or *vascul/o*.

6: There are two combining forms that appear in words referring to the blood vessels. This is one of many cases in health sciences terminology in which you must learn by experience which form to use when building specific words. For example, use the shorter combining form to build the word that means "the excision of part or all of a blood vessel." *Vasectomy*

vas/ectomy

7: Now use the longer combining form to build a word that refers to the heart and the blood vessels (and note the

51

cardi/o/vascul

adjective suffix) _Cardiovascular_

8: A disease or abnormality of both the blood vessels and the nervous system is called vas/o/ _neurolopathy_

neur/o/path/y

9: The combining form that refers to the liver is *hepat/o*. You know the word *hepat/itis* refers to the liver when you see the word root _hepat_ .

hepat

liver

10: The word *hepat/algia* means "pain in the _liver_ ."

11: A disease or abnormality of the liver is called _hepatopathy_ .

hepat/o/path/y

12: Build a word that means "pertaining to both the liver and the stomach" (and watch your suffix) _hepatogastric_

hepat/o/gastr/ic

13: A *hernia* is the protrusion of a body part from its natural cavity. The word part *-cele*, a suffix, means "hernia." Build a word that means "a protrusion of liver tissue from its natural cavity." _hepatocele_

hepat/o/cele

14: You know that the word *encephal/o/cele* means "a protrusion of brain tissue from its natural cavity" when you see the word part _hepatocele_

cele

15: A protrusion of a section of the intestine from its natural cavity is an _enterocele_.

enter/o/cele

16: The word part that refers to the bladder is *cyst/o*. Build a word that means "a hernia (Remember Question 13?) of the bladder." _cystocele_

cyst/o/cele

17: In building words referring to the bladder, use the combining form *cyst/o* or a form of it. Use the *-ic* adjective suffix to build a word that means "pertaining to both the liver and the bladder." _hepatocystic_

hepat/o/cyst/ic

cystitis

18: An inflammation of the bladder is called: _____ .

19: A surgical operation in which an incision is made into the bladder for drainage (a more or less "permanent" opening) is called a _cystostomy_. (Think carefully about definitions.)

cystostomy

20: The suffix *-plasty* refers to the surgical formation or repair of a body part. In the word *cyst/o/plasty*, the word part that means "surgical repair" is _plasty_ .

plasty

21: The word *rhin/o/plasty* means "a surgical repair of the nose." In this and many other health sciences terms, the suffix -plasty and related forms always mean _surgical formation_

surgical formation
  or repair

22: A *mastectomy* (mast/o + ectomy) is a surgical removal of the breast sometimes made necessary by such diseases as cancer of the breast. Following such an operation, it may be possible to surgically build up tissues to repair the appearance of the breast. Draw a conclusion: Such a

mast/o/plasty

surgical repair is called *mastoplasty*

23: Build a word that means "a surgical repair of the

enter/o/plasty

intestine." *enteroplasty*

24: The combining form *splen/o* refers to the spleen. In words that refer to the spleen, you should use some form of

splen/o

splen/o .

splen/otomy

25: A surgical incision of the spleen is called a *splenotomy*

26: Look carefully! A general term for a tumor of the spleen

splenoma

is *splenoma*. However, a specific two-word term for

splen/ic

a cancerous neoplasm of the spleen is *splenic*

carcinoma.

27: Therapy is the general term that means "treatment designed to eliminate disease or other body disorder." You may describe almost any kind of treatment of a

therapy

disease or body disorder as *therapy*

28: Treatment of a body disorder that employs physical

therapy

agents or methods is called physical *therapy*

29: The adjective *therapeutic* means "pertaining to the treatment of a disease or other body disorder." A drug administered to counteract some specific disease, then, is

therapeutic

a *therapeutic* drug.

30: Sometimes a word for a specific kind of therapy is built by using a combining form. In the word *chem/o/therapy* (meaning "treatment by means of chemical agents"), the

therapy

word meaning "treatment" is *therapy*

chem/o

The word part meaning "chemical" is *chemo* .

31: The treatment of a disorder of the nervous system can be

neur/o/therapy

called *neurotherapy*.

32: The word *therapeutic* may also refer to the effect of therapy. The application of an antibiotic to disease-

therapeutic

causing (pathogenic) microorganisms may have a *therapeutic*

effect.

33: The prefix *ortho-* means "straight," "normal," or "correct." When building words that refer to a straight, normal, or correct condition, you will often use the prefix

ortho

ortho .

orth

34: The word part *optic* relates to vision. Use the correct prefix to build a word meaning "normal vision." (Think about avoiding a double vowel here.) _Orth/optic_

(Did that one throw you? If so, remember that most health sciences terms avoid double vowels when joining two word parts.)

orth/odont

35: Use a form of odont/o (tooth) to build a word meaning "the dental specialty that deals with the maintenance of straight teeth." _Orth/odont/ics_

ortho/cephal/ic

36: Use the *-ic* adjective suffix to build a word meaning "normal skull" (a skull height that is normal). _Ortho/cephal/ic_

37: The combining form *megal/o* means "enlarged" or "large." (Remember macr/o?) The word *megal/o/gastr/ia* means "enlarged stomach," so the part of the word that

megal/o

means "large" is _megal/o_.

38: Various forms of *megal/o* may appear at different places within the whole word. For instance, in the word *acr/o/megal/y* (meaning "enlarged extremities") the word

enlarged or large

part *megal/y* appears at the end and means _large_.

39: Only experience will teach you which words require *megal/o* at the beginning and which at the end. The word

megal/y
megal/o

for enlargement of the intestine is enter/o/ _megal_. But the word for enlarged heart is _megal/o_ cardi/a.

40: Whenever you see a form of *megal/o*, you should think of

large

large.

41: The combining form *muc/o* refers to mucus. Whenever

mucus

you see some form of muc/o, you should think of _mucus_

42: *Mucus* is secreted by the mucous membranes. Note the difference in spelling in the two words. The word root for

muc

both words is _muc_.

43: Another word for mucous membrane is *mucosa*. Mucus is

mucosa

secreted by the _mucosa_.

44: Certain tissues and fluids of the body resemble mucus, but are not mucus. You would describe such tissues and fluids

muc/oid

with the term _muc/oid_

mucosa, or
mucous membrane

45: Mucus is secreted by the _mucosa_ , or _mucous membrane_.

There are some body substances that resemble mucus;

mucoid

they are called _mucoid_ .

46: Try a quick review. The combining form meaning "heart" is _Cardio_ . The combining form meaning "spleen" is _spleno_ . The combining form meaning "bladder" is _cysto_ .

cardi/o
splen/o
cyst/o

47: The word part _chole_- refers to bile, but when it is joined to the word part meaning "bladder" it forms a word meaning "gallbladder." Form the word that means "gallbladder." _Chole/cyst_

chole/cyst

48: Use the word parts _chole_-, _cyst/o_, and the correct suffix to build a word meaning "pain in the gallbladder." _Chole/cyst/algia_

chole/cyst/algia

49: Even though it is made up of parts with their own individual meanings, cholecyst has a whole meaning (gallbladder) of its own. Build a word that means "a removal of part or all of the gallbladder." _Cholecyst/ectomy_

cholecyst/ectomy

50: _Cholecyst/o_ is the combining form of cholecyst. Now build a word that means "the making of a new opening between the gallbladder and the duodenum." _Cholecyst/o/duoden/ostomy_

cholecyst/o/
duoden/ostomy

(After successfully completing that word-building assignment, you deserve congratulations.)

51: The combining form _lith/o_ means "stone." In the word _chole/lith_, the word part that means "stone" is _lith_.

lith

52: A chole/lith is produced in the chole/cyst. Chole means _gall_ . Cyst means _bladder_ . Lith means _stone_ .

gall (bile); bladder
stone

53: As you no doubt remember, the combining form _rhin/o_ refers to the nose. Build a word meaning "a stone, or calcification, in the nose." _rhinolith_

rhin/o/lith

54: The surgical removal of a gallstone is called a _Cholelithectomy_

chole/lith/ectomy

55: Using the combining form for heart and the longer word root for blood vessel, build an adjective that means "pertaining to both the heart and the blood vessels." _Cardiovascular_

cardi/o/vascul/ar
hepat/o
enterocele

56: The combining form for liver is _hepatio_ .
57: A hernia of the intestine, called an _enterocele_, is often treated by surgical repair of the intestine, an operation called _enteroplasty_

enteroplasty

therapy

58: The treatment of a cancerous growth by administering a chemical agent designed to eliminate the cancer is called cancer chem/o/ *therapy*

normal

59: In the word *orthography*, the prefix ortho- means *normal*

60: The word that means "enlargement of the spleen" is

megal/y

splen/o/ *megaly*

You have completed Unit 7. Look over your work carefully. You may work through the entire unit again, if you feel you need to do so.

REVIEW LIST

This list of words is for your personal review. The number beside each word indicates the question in Unit 7 in which you began learning that word or word part. Space is provided for you to make notes for review.

cardi/o (1) *heart*

vas/o, vascul/o (5) *blood vessel*

hepat/o (9) *liver*

-cele (13) *hernia*

cyst/o (16) *bladder*

-plasty (20) *surgical repair*

splen/o (24) *spleen*

therapy (27) *treatment*

ortho (33) *normal*

megal/o (37) *enlarged*

muc/o (41) *mucus*

chole, cholecyst (47) *gall bladder*

lith/o (51) *stone*

UNIT 8

Directions: In this unit you are going to be asked to think very carefully and to solve some rather difficult word-building problems. Don't despair. You're doing very well so far, and you shouldn't have any real trouble with the terms in this unit. Use your cover card.

1: To review, build a word that means "a surgical operation to make a new pathway (or communication) between the gallbladder and the stomach."

cholecyst/o/
gastr/ostomy

cholecyst o gastrostomy

2: The combining form *narc/o* means "relating to stupor" and is used in building words that refer to sleep or to numbness. Narc/o often appears in words relating to sedation. As you learned in Unit 2, the suffix *-osis* means "a condition of the body or body part." Build a word that means "a (bodily) condition of stupor or numbness."

narc/osis

narc o osis

3: If the word *narc/o/tic* means "a drug that induces sleep or stupor," which part of the word refers to sleep?

narc/o

narc o

4: In Unit 2 you learned that therapy administered to relieve pain is called *analgesic*. What two-word term would you use to describe therapy that relieves pain by inducing sleep or stupor?

narcotic analgesic

narcotic analgesic

5: Do not confuse analgesia (lacking sensitivity to pain) with *anesthesia* (lacking sensitivity to all sensation or stimuli). If pain exists, you would administer an an/ _alges_ /ic.

alges

To prevent pain, and all other sensations, you would administer an an/ _esthe_ /tic.

esthe

(That was a tricky one. If you built the correct words, or came close, you're doing well.)

6: If *an/esthes/ia* means "lacking sensitivity to sensation or stimuli," what part of the word refers to sensitivity to sensation or stimuli? _esthes_

esthes

57

an/esthes/i/ology

7: Now build a word that means "the study of the lack of sensitivity to sensation or stimuli." *anesthesiology*

8: The word meaning "one who studies lack of sensitivity to sensation or stimuli" also names the M.D. who administers anesthetic in the operating room. Build the word.
an / esthes /i/ ologist

an/esthes/i/ologist

analgesic

9: Once more: an agent (drug or other therapy) that *relieves* pain is an *analgesic* .
An agent that *prevents* pain by creating a lack of sensitivity to sensation or stimuli is an *anesthetic*
An agent that produces a state of stupor or sleepiness is a *narcotic*.

anesthetic

narcotic

10: The combining form *radi/o* is used in building words that refer to the emission of electromagnetic energy in certain forms; this emission is usually referred to as radioactivity. In building words that refer to radioactivity, you should use the combining form *radio* .

radi/o

11: Radioactivity has many applications in health care, in both diagnosis and therapy. Use the correct form of *radi/o* to build a word that means "the study of radioactivity."
radi /ology

radi/ology

12: The word part *gram* means "written," but it may also refer to any recording of information. Use gram as a suffix in building a word that means "a recorded picture of internal body structures made by using radioactivity."
radio/gram

radi/o/gram

radi/o/encephal/o/gram

13: Now build a word that specifically means "a picture of the brain recorded by using radioactivity."
radio/encephalo gram

14: Build a word meaning "the treatment of a disease or body disorder by use of radioactivity." *radiotherapy*

radi/o/therapy

15: The prefix *con-* means "with." It appears in a great many health sciences terms. In the word *contaminate* (meaning "to soil with infectious material"), what part of the word means "with"? *con*

con

16: If a sterile or aseptic dressing is exposed to infectious bacteria, the bacteria may *contaminate* the dressing.

contaminate

17: When *duct* is used as a word part, it refers to movement. *Con/duct/ion* refers to the *movement* of energy or matter.

movement

18: The term *conduction* is often used to refer to neuromuscular activity. The neuromuscular impulses that are
normal in heart function are called cardiac *Conduction*

conduction

19: The process by which activating impulses are transmitted
from nerve to muscle fiber, and then from muscle fiber to
other muscle fiber within the heart, is called *Cardiac
Conduction*.

cardiac
conduction

20: Do not confuse *con*duction with *in*duction. *Induction* is
generally the process of causing or producing. When a
change in one body part causes a change in another body
part nearby, the process is called *induction*

induction

21: An enzyme is a substance, secreted within the body, that
causes certain chemical changes to take place. The action
of an enzyme in causing change may be called enzyme
induction

induction

22: When energy or matter is transmitted, the process is called
Conduction.

conduction

When some change is caused or some effect is produced,
the process is called *induction*

induction

23: The prefix *epi-* means "upon." In the word *epidermis*,
meaning "the outer layer of skin" ("upon the skin"),
which word part means "upon"? *epi*

epi

24: An inflammation of the outer layer of skin is called
epi/dermat/*itis*.

epi/ /itis

25: The word *cranium* is commonly used to mean "the skull."
By adding the correct prefix, you can build a word that
means "the layers of muscle and skin which cover, or are
upon, the skull." *epi/cranium*

epi/cranium

26: A disease in which the patient is subject to unconscious-
ness or convulsions is described by a term that literally
means "seizure upon." If the word part *-lepsy* means
seizure, what word means seizure upon? *epilepsy*

epi/lepsy

27: Many words come from the Greek word *demos*, meaning
"people." A disease that attacks, or comes upon, many
people simultaneously is an *epi*/dem/ic.

epi

28: Now build a word that means "the study of disease which
attacks many people simultaneously." *epidemiology*

epi/dem/ /ology

29: Whenever you see the prefix *epi-*, you should think of
upon.

upon

30: The word part *blast* means "an immature or unformed

tumor, or neoplasm
immature cell

cell." In the term *blastoma* -oma means ___*tumor*___
and blast means ___*immature cell*___

31: Whenever you see *blast* as a word part, you should think of an immature cell. How would you define *erythroblast*?
___*an immature blood cell*___

an immature red
  blood cell

32: You can now define *leukoblastosis* as ___*abnormal*___
___*condition of the white blood cells*___

an abnormal condition
  of the immature
  white blood cells

33: When used as a prefix, *mal-* means "bad" or "incorrect." Whenever you see the prefix mal-, think of ___*bad*___
or ___*incorrect*___ .

bad
incorrect

34: The word *occlusion* means "closure," so the dental condition in which the teeth do not close correctly is called a ___*mal occulsion*___

mal/occlusion
incorrect

35: *Malabsorption* is ___*incorrect*___ absorption.

36: Do not confuse words with *mal-* as a prefix with words in which mal is the first syllable, even though meanings may sometimes be the same. The word *malacia*, which means "an abnormal softening of tissue," may denote an "incorrect" condition, but you should not consider the first syllable a prefix. Instead, whenever you see the word, malacia, you should think of ___*an abnormal*___ ___*softening of tissue*___

an abnormal softening
  of tissue

37: Sometimes *malacia* is used as a suffix that refers to an abnormal softening of tissue. In the word *oste/o/malacia*, oste/o refers to ___*bone*___ and malacia refers to ___*an abnormal softening*___

bone
an abnormal softening
  of tissue

38: When you see the combining form *malac/o*, you know that the word root that refers to abnormal softening of tissue is ___*malac*___ .

malac

39: Now build a word that means "an abnormal softening of brain tissue." ___*Encephalomalac*___ia.

encephal/o/malac

40: What word means "a surgical excision, or removal, of softened tissue"? ___*malac/ectomy*___

malac/ectomy

41: Oste/o/arthr/o/path/y is a word meaning "a disease of the bones and joints." *Arthr/o* is a combining form that refers to the ___*joints*___ .

joints

42: For the sake of review, analyze the word oste/o/arthr/o/path/y:

oste/o

arthr/o

path

y

arthr/itis

arthromalacia

ather

ather/o

atherosclerosis

arteri/o/sclerosis

arteri/o/path/y

arteriectomy

arterioplasty
arteriomalacia
sleep, or
stupor

epi/derm/al

alges
esthes

oste/o is the combining form for bone

arthr/o is the combining form for joint

path is the word root for disease

_y_ is the noun ending

43: Inflammation that occurs in a joint is called _arthr itis_

44: When the tissue of a joint begins to soften, you refer to the condition as _arthromalacia_

45: You should not confuse arthr/o with words that contain athero-. _Athero-_ refers to inorganic fatty matter, which may collect and form obstructions in some body parts. In the word _ather/oma_, the word part that refers to fatty matter is _ather_ .

46: The word _sclerosis_ means "a hardening of tissue." When a hardening of the arteries is accompanied by deposits of fatty matter, the condition is called _athero_ sclerosis.

47: A disease in which blood circulation through the body is obstructed by hardening of and fatty deposits in the arteries is called _atherosclerosis_

48: Do not confuse athero-, which refers to inorganic fatty matter, with the combining form _arteri/o_, which refers to the arteries. (The arteries are the vessels that carry oxygenated blood _to_ the body; veins carry blood _from_ the body to the heart and lungs.) Use the combining form arteri/o to build a word that means only "hardening of the arteries." _arteri/o sclerosis_

49: With your newfound knowledge of arteri/o, build a word that means "a disease of the arteries." _arterio pathy_

50: Sometimes disease may make the excision of part or all of an artery necessary. This operation is an _arteriectomy_ Following this operation, surgical repair or replacement of the artery may be possible. This surgical repair is called _arterioplasty_.

51: Softening of an arterial wall is _arteriomalacia_

52: Words containing some form of _narc/o_ refer to _sleep_ _stupor_ .

53: Use the _-al_ adjective ending to build a word that means "relating to the outer layer of skin." _epidermal_

54: Supply the missing word parts:
an/_alges_/ic, pain-relieving agent
an/_esthes_/ia, lacking sensitivity to stimuli

arthr
arteri
athero

arth/o/plasty, surgical repair of a joint
arteri/o/gram, radiogram of an artery
ather/genesis, production of inorganic fatty matter

You have completed Unit 8. Look over your work carefully. You may work through the entire unit again, if you feel you need to do so.

Unit 8 is one of the most difficult units in the program—so far. If you worked through this unit, learned some new terms, and retained your sense of humor, you have done a commendable job.

REVIEW LIST

This list of words is for your personal review. The number beside each word indicates the question in Unit 8 in which you began learning that word or word part. Space is provided for you to make notes for review.

narc/o (2)   *Sleep*

anesthesia, anesthetic (5)

radi/o (10)

conduction (15)

induction (20)

epi- (23)

epidemic (27)

blast (30)

mal- (33)

malac/o (36)

arthr/o (41)

ather/o (45)

sclerosis (46)

arteri/o (48)

Review Test for Units 7 & 8

Directions: This review test covers the words and word parts learned in Units 7 and 8. *This is NOT a test to be graded.* It is for your use only. Since the review tests in this program are designed to help you check your learning progress, you should make as much use of them as possible. If your work on this review test doesn't satisfy you, for example, why not work through Units 7 and 8 again? Then repeat the review test. The object of self-instruction is to learn, not to beat the clock. The answers are on page 65.

1: Define cardiovascular radiogram as concisely as possible.
An Xray of the heart and blood vessels by the use of radiography —

2: A surgical operation that creates a new opening or pathway between the liver and the stomach is called a *hep a to gastric ostomy*

3: If you examined an X-ray and found evidence of an encephalocele, what would you be seeing? *A hernia of the brain area*

4: Build the words that match the following definitions:

   a) surgical repair of the intestine *enter /o/ plast / y*

   b) dental specialty that deals with the maintenance of "straight, or correct, teeth"
   Ortho /dont/ ia

   c) new opening between the gallbladder and the duodenum
   Cholecyst /o/ duoden / ostomy

   d) surgical removal of a gallstone *chol /lith / ectomy*

   e) condition of stupor or sleepiness *narc /o/ osis*

5: A patient who is suffering pain would be administered an _analgesic_ to relieve the pain. A patient who is being prepared for a pain-producing operation would be administered an _anesthetic_ to prevent the pain.

6: Arthritis can be described as _an inflammation_ in a _joint_.

7: Break down the following terms into their component parts (word roots, combining forms, prefixes, and suffixes) and define each component part.

Term	Parts	Definitions
epidemiology	epi	upon
	demi	people
	olog	study
	y	noun ending
leukoblastosis	leuko	white
	blast	immature cell
	osis	abnormal condition
arteriomalacia	arteri	arteries
	malac	softening
	ia	noun ending
cystoid	cyst	bladder
	oid	like
vasoneuropathy	vaso	vessels
	neuro	nerves
	path	disease
	y	noun ending

You have completed the review test for Units 7 and 8. Go over your work until you are satisfied that you have done your best. Then check your answers with the answers on page 65. If you have any incorrect answers on this test, correct them at once. But leave a mark by those items which you missed, so that you may refer to them again.

ANSWERS: UNITS 7 & 8

1. a picture or recording (gram) of the heart (cardi/o) and blood vessels (vascul/ar) by use of radioactivity (radi/o)

2. hepat/o/gastr/ostomy

3. a hernia, or protrusion from its natural cavity, of brain tissue

4. a) enter/o/plast/y
    b) orth/odont/ics
    c) cholecyst/o/duoden/ostomy
    d) chole/lith/ectomy
    e) narc/osis

5. analgesic; anesthetic

6. inflammation in a joint

7.

Term	Parts	Definitions
epidemiology	epi	upon
	dem(i)	people
	olog	study
	y	noun ending
leukoblastosis	leuk/o	white
	blast	immature cell
	osis	abnormal condition
arteriomalacia	arteri/o	arteries
	malac	softening
	ia	noun ending
cystoid	cyst	bladder
	oid	resembling or like
vasoneuropathy	vas/o	vessels
	neur/o	nerves, or nervous system
	path	disease
	y	noun ending

UNIT 9

Directions: Unit 9, like all those preceding it, calls for the use of your cover card.

carrier

1: In the field of epidemiology, you will study the carrier. The *carrier* is an individual, not necessarily human, who carries disease organisms in his body. In working to control some epidemics, health officials must locate the _*Carrier*_ who is carrying disease organisms in his body.

symptoms

2: A carrier, although carrying a disease, shows no symptoms of the disease. It is difficult to locate a carrier, because he shows no _*symptoms*_ of the disease he is carrying.

carrier

3: A human or animal who carries disease organisms in his body and infects others while showing no symptoms himself is called a _*carrier*_.

path/o/gen

4: An organism that produces disease is called a _*pathogenic*_ organism.

disease-producing or pathogenic, organisms

5: The *coccus* bacteria are a family of disease-producing organisms. Whenever you see coccus, or its plural cocci, you will know the word refers to a family of _*disease producing*_.

cocc

6: The word root of cocc/us and cocc/i is _*cocc*_.

cocc/i

7: Pneumonia is caused by the pneumococcus. The bacteria that cause pneumonia belong to the _*cocci*_ (plural) family.

cocc/i

cocc/i

cocc/i

8: Bacteriologists are familiar with three main types of cocci. Cocci that grow in pairs are called dipl/o/_*cocci*_. Cocci growing in twisted chains are called strept/o/_*cocci*_. Cocci growing in clusters like grapes are called staphyl/o/_*cocci*_.

strept/o

strept/o/cocc/us

staphyl/o/cocc/i

staphyl/o/cocc/i

dipl/o/cocc/us

strept/o/cocc/us

dipl/o

staphyl/itis

pro

pro

pro/gnosis

9: Strept/o is from a Greek word meaning "twisted." If you examine a slide of cocci and see what looks like a twisted chain, you can identify the organism as ~~strept~~/cocc/i.

10: *Strept/o/dermat/itis* is an inflammation of the skin caused by the ~~streptococcus~~ (singular) bacterium.

11: *Staphyl/o* is from the Greek word meaning "a bunch of grapes." Staphyl/o is used to build words that refer to structures that resemble bunches of grapes. Cocci that grow in clusters resembling bunches of grapes are ~~staphylococci~~.

12: A *carbuncle* is a draining skin sore caused by cocci that grow in a cluster. Carbuncles are caused by ~~staphylococci~~.

13: The coccus organism that grows in pairs is the ~~diplococcus~~.

A sore throat may be a symptom of an infection caused by a coccus that grows in a twisted-chain formation, the ~~streptococcus~~.

A tissue that is formed of two layers of immature cells is described as ~~dipl/o~~/blast/ic. (Think!)

The structure that hangs in the back of the mouth like a bunch of grapes (open your mouth and look in a mirror if you don't believe it) is the *uvula*. In building words that refer to the uvula, you should use the combining form that means "a bunch of grapes." So the word that means "inflammation of the uvula" is ~~staphylitis~~

(Good thinking! Keep at it.)

14: The prefix *pro-* means "coming before," "in front of," or "in favor of." It is often used as the opposite of anti-. In building words that refer to coming before, in front of, or in favor of, use the prefix ~~pro~~.

15: *Projection* means "extending in front of." The word part that means "in front of" is ~~pro~~.

16: You have learned that the word *dia/gnosis* means "know completely." Use the correct prefix to build a word meaning "know before." ~~pro gnosis~~.

17: After a diagnosis has been made, a physician is often able to "predict" the course of a disease and its probable outcome. He can be said to "know before" the results of pro/gnosis

an attack by disease. This knowing before is called a
prog thosis

18: The word *pro/phylaxis* means "preventing disease." The word part phylaxis comes from a Greek word meaning "to guard"; the literal meaning, then, of pro/phylaxis is "to

before

guard *before* ."

19: The adjective form of pro/phylaxis is *pro/phylactic*. Any agent that acts to prevent disease can be described as

pro/phylactic

pro/phylactic.

20: Do not confuse the prefix *pro-* with the syllable pro in such words as protein. Also, watch out for such forms as *pros* in the word pros/thesis, which means "the replacement of a lost body part with an artificial one." *Pros/thesis* is compounded of Greek derivatives literally meaning "an addition." When speaking of the "addition" of an artificial part to the body, you will often use the

pros/thesis

word *pros thesis*

21: Although *prosth* is not a recognized word root, it appears in nearly all words that refer to artificial body parts. Build a word that means "the science of constructing and fitting

prosth

artificial dental appliances." *Prosth*odontics.

prosthesis

22: The use of an artificial eye or lens is called ocular *prosthesis*

23: The combining form that means "eye" is *ocul/o*. A word that means "pertaining to the eyes and face" is

ocul/o

ocul/o/faci/al.

24: *Ocul/o/motor* is an adjective that means "pertaining to

ocul/o
motor

eye movement." In this word, *ocul o* means "eye" and *motor* refers to movement.

25: *Ot/o* is the combining form that means "ear." Just for fun, build a word (not medically recognized) that means "pertaining to the unusual ear movement called wiggling."

ot/o
ot/o
log/y

ot/o/motor

26: In the word *otology*, *ot/o* means "ear" and *log/y* means "the study of."

27: *Orrhea* is a combining form that often appears as a suffix meaning "flow" or "discharge." Use orrhea to build a

ot/orrhea

word meaning "a discharge from the ear." *ot/orrhea*

28: The condition that you described by building a word in Question 27 is often a symptom of an ear inflammation.

ot/itis

called *ot/itis* .

rhin/orrhea

29: The combining form that means "nose" is *rhin/o*. What word would describe a flow or discharge from the nose? *rhin orrhea*

rhin/o/plast/y

30: The word root *rhin* and the combining form *rhin/o* refer to the nose as a facial structure. Surgery to repair the structure of the nose is called *rhin o plasty* .

rhin/o/lith

31: Now build a word that means "a stone or calcification located in the nose." *rhin o lith*

32: *Laryng/o* is the combining form that means "the throat" generally or, specifically, "the larynx." In building words about the larynx (where the vocal chords are located), use

laryng/o

some form of ___ *laryng o* ___ .

laryng/itis

33: Severe hoarseness is often a symptom of an inflammation of the larynx, called ___ *laryngitis* ___ .

laryng/ectomy

34: A carcinoma in the larynx may necessitate excision of the vocal chords. This operation is called a ___ *laryngectomy*

35: The last 10 questions have prepared you to build a word which is the name of a medical specialty that is the study of the ear, nose, and throat. Build this word. ___ *ot o*

ot/o/
rhin/o/laryng/o/log/y

rhino laryngalogy

(It is a pleasure to point out that you are making excellent progress as a student of health sciences terminology. Of course, it is sometimes difficult to work otorhinolaryngology into a conversation—unless you are talking with an otorhinolaryngologist. But your ability to build such a word is a good measure of the progress you are making in learning the elements of all health sciences terminology.)

36: The word parts *metric* and *metry* are both related to the suffix *-meter*, which refers to an instrument for measuring. A *cardi/o/meter* is an instrument that measures the power of the heart action. When you see or hear the suffix

instrument

-meter, you should think of an *instrument* for measuring.

37: As you learned in Unit 4, *bi/o* is the combining form that means "life." Since *-metry* refers to the process of measuring, the word that means "the process of measuring

metry

statistically the effects of biological facts" is bi/o/ *metry.*

38: Biostatistics is the area of health science that deals with masses of data concerning human life activities—birth and death rates, disease data, and so on. What part of the word *biostatistics* tells you that life is involved in the meaning?

bio
bio

39: The word part *graph* refers to a recording, as do the related word parts *-graphy*, *-graphic*, and *-gram*. The recording of a person's life is called a bi/o/_graphy_ .

graphy

40: The combining form *dem/o* comes from the Greek word for people, so the science that deals with recording the health and other characteristics of a large unit of people is called dem/o/_graphy_

graphy

41: The form *-gram* usually refers to the recorded form (a chart, an X-ray photograph, or the like) produced in *-graphic* recording. *Electr/o/cardi/o/graphy* measures and records the electrical activity of the heart. The recorded form produced by electrocardiography is an _electro cardio gram_

electr/o/cardi/o/gram

42: The suffix *-graph* refers to the instrument that does the recording. An *electr/o/cardi/o/gram* is produced by an instrument called an _electro cardio graph_

electr/o/cardi/o/graph

43: In the word *demography*, the suffix *-graphy* refers to the science of recording the health and other characteristics of _people_ .

people

In the word electroencephalogram,
electr/o refers to _electric_
encephal/o refers to _the brain_
-gram is a _recorded form_

electric activity
the brain
recorded form

44: Build a word meaning "the science or process of recording the electrical activity of the stomach." _electro gastro graphy_

electr/o/gastr/o/graphy

45: Remember this difference: a cardi/o/meter is an instrument that _measures_ heart activity; a cardi/o/graph is an instrument that _records_ heart activity.

measures
records

46: A human or animal who carries infectious disease organisms in his body while not being infected himself is called a _carrier_

carrier

47: Cocci that grow in pairs are _diplococci_ . Cocci growing in twisted chains are _streptococci_ . Cocci growing in clusters like grapes are _staphylococci_

diplococci
streptococci
staphylococci

48: The word *prosthesis* means "an _artificial_ body part."

artificial

49: Build a word meaning "a flow or discharge from the larynx." _laryngorrhea_

laryng/orrhea

excellent

50: Anyone who has learned all these health science terms is making excellent progress in this program. Since you have learned a great many terms, you are making *excellent* progress.

You have completed Unit 9. Look over your work carefully.

R E V I E W   L I S T

This list of words is for your personal review. The number beside each word indicates the question in Unit 9 in which you began learning that word or word part. Space is provided for you to make notes for review.

carrier (1)	**ocul/o** (23)
cocc/us (5)	**ot/o** (25)
dipl/o (8)	**orrhea** (27)
strept/o (9)	**rhin/o** (29)
staphyl/o (11)	**laryng/o** (32)
pro- (14)	**-meter, -metry** (36)
prosthesis (20)	**graph, -graphy, -gram** (39)

UNIT 10

Directions: The method of working through this final unit in health sciences terminology is the same as in all the preceding units: use your cover card and work conscientiously. Also, as in all preceding units, you are the only one who profits or who does not profit from your work. And you are the only one who can know with certainty how much you are learning from this program.

1: To review, a microscopic examination of a slide shows bacteria growing in clusters like bunches of grapes means

staphyl/o   that the slide contains _staphylococc/i_.

prosthesis   The general term that means "an artificial body part" is _prosthesis_.

cardiometer   An instrument that *measures* the activity of the heart is a _cardio·meter_.

cardiograph   An instrument that *records* the activity of the heart is a _cardiograph_.

2: The combining form *physi/o* is used in words that refer to the functions of various parts and organs of living

physi/o   organisms. In the word *physi/o/log/y*, _physi/o_ refers to the functions of living organisms.

3: Sometimes the term *physical therapy* is written as one word, making use of the combining form that refers to the functions of various parts and organs of a living organism.

physi/o   Can you build that word? _physi/o/_therapy

4: Do not confuse *physi/o* (referring to the physical functions of organisms) with *psych/o* (referring to the mind).

physi/o   Remember that _physi/o_/log/y is a study of physical func-
psych/o   tions, whereas _psych/o_/log/y is a study of mental functions.

5: Now build a word that means "the production of mental

psych/o/genesis   functions." _psych/o/genesis_

73

psych/osis

6: Recall the correct suffix to build a word meaning "an abnormal condition of the mental functions." ____/____

7: The combining form *my/o* is used in building words that refer to muscle. In the word *my/o/path/y* (a disease or dysfunction of the muscles), the word part referring to muscle is ____/____ .

my/o

my/o/plast/y
relating to both
    muscle and nerve

8: Use the correct suffix to build the word meaning "surgical repair of muscle tissue." ____/__/____/____

9: Can you define the term myoneural? _____
_____

10: Do not confuse *my/o* with *myc/o*, the combining form that means "fungus." Remember that my/o/log/y is the study of _____ , but myc/o/log/y is the study of _____ .

muscle
fungus

11: The condition known as *myc/o/gastr/itis* is an inflammation of the mucous membrane of the stomach caused by a _____ .

fungus

guards
    against fungus

12: *Mycophylaxin* is the name of a substance that _____
_____

(Look at the word parts carefully.)

myc/osis

13: Any abnormal condition (such as a disease) that is caused by fungus is called a ____/____ .

14: You have learned that my/o refers to muscle and myc/o refers to fungus. To keep your mind sharp, remember that *myel/o* refers either to bone marrow or the spinal cord. So make a mental checklist:

muscle
fungus
bone marrow or
    spinal cord

my/o is _____
myc/o is _____
myel/o is _____ or _____

cell

15: You will usually be able to tell whether myel/o refers to bone marrow or to the spinal cord by the context in which it appears. For instance, a *myel/o/cyte* is a _____ in bone marrow.

16: Since it is difficult to imagine a hernia of bone marrow, you can probably assume that *myelocele* is a hernia of the _____ .

spinal cord

17: An abnormal or pathologic hardening of the spinal cord is called _____/__/_____ . The same kind of hardening of muscle tissue would be called ____/__/____ .

myel/o/sclerosis
my/o/sclerosis

my/o
myc/o
myel/o

18: Once again:

    ____/___ is the combining form for muscle

    ____/___ is the combining form for fungus

    _____/___ is the combining form for spinal cord or bone marrow

(Good job!)

19: You have already learned that the forms derma and dermat/o are used in building words referring to the skin. The word *cutaneous* also pertains to the skin. So the word

skin

*sub*cutaneous means "below the _____ ."

20: The word *subcutaneous* is used to refer to body tissues

below the skin

that are _____.

21: Think carefully! A disease caused by fungus located in the tissues below the skin might be described as _____

subcutaneous
  mycopathy

_____ (two words).

hypodermic

22: An injection administered just under the skin is a _____ injection.

(Confusing? Don't worry. Experience in using words will get you into the habit of using the right one in the right context.)

23: You have learned that the prefix sub- means "below," as do the prefixes hypo- and infra-. Another much-used prefix is *ex-*, meaning "from" or "out of." If the word

ex

tension literally means to stretch, then _____/tension is the stretching of a limb into a straightened position.

24: An *ex/crescence* is any outgrowth from the surface, usually a tissue surface. The part of this word that means

ex
from
out of

"out of" is_____ .

25: An *ex/tended* limb is one that is stretched _____ or _____ a flexed position.

26: The prefix *dys-* means "bad" or "difficult." So a muscular

bad or difficult

dys/function is a _____ or _____ functioning of muscle tissue

bad or
  difficult intestine

27: When broken into its component parts, *dys/enter/y* means _____ .

28: The word that means "an impaired (bad or difficult) nerve

dys/neur

function" is _____/_____/ia.

29: Look carefully at the word *dysosteogenesis*. Now define

incorrect (bad)
  bone formation

it. _____
_____

trans

30: The prefix *trans-* means "across," "through," or "beyond." Anything that passes through the chest cavity could be described as _____ /thoracic.

31: Absorption is one way in which a substance may pass through the skin without breaking it. A process by which substances pass through unbroken skin may be described

trans/cutaneous
trans/dermic

as either _____ /_____ or _____ /_____ .

trans/ocul

32: Anything that moves or grows across the eye could be described as _____ /_____ /ar.

(The next few questions are a bit different from the ones so far. You will read a few sentences and then fill in the answers with your understanding of the sentences you've read.

Neurofibroma is a physiological condition. It may occur in the form of dermatoma, osteoma, or intestinal neoplasm. One type of neurofibroma may involve a myelosis.

physical

33: The condition referred to is a _____ (physical, mental) disorder.

physi/o

What word part(s) tells you this? _____

34: The condition referred to does not involve which of the following? (Check one)

____ (a) the nervous system
____ (b) a tumorous growth

(c) the gallbladder

____ (c) the gallbladder
____ (d) fibrous tissue

35: The condition referred to may occur in all the following tissues but one. Check the tissue it does not occur in.

____ (a) the spinal cord

(b) a tooth socket

____ (b) a tooth socket
____ (c) bone tissue
____ (d) skin
____ (e) intestinal tissue

An *anticoagulant* may be the indicated chemotherapy in some cases of atherosclerosis. In extreme cases, however, procedures ranging from peripheral vasectomy to arteriectomy may be necessary.

36: The condition referred to involves all but which one of the following?

____ (a) the veins and arteries
____ (b) inorganic fatty deposits

_____ (c) a hardening process

_____ _____ (d) the joints

(d) the joints

chemical

37: The primary therapy referred to involves _____
(physical, chemical) agents.

38: In extreme cases, which treatment is *not* referred to?

(a) making a new
opening in the
periodontium

_____ (a) making a new opening in the periodontium

_____ (b) excising parts of arteries

_____ (c) excising parts of blood vessels

An ambulatory ward is not the best place to research the etiology of certain pathogenic conditions. If the patient is allowed to ambulate, maintaining asepsis over his whole body is impossible, although standard prophylactic measures should be taken.

causes

disease

39: The passage refers to researching the _____ of
_____-producing conditions.

40: The ward referred to is one for patients who are able to

walk, or move about

_____ .

guard against or
prevent infection

41: The passage says that measures should be taken to _____
_____ .

42: The passage says that it is impossible to maintain (check
one)

_____ (a) watchfulness over the patient

(b) freedom from
infection

_____ (b) freedom from infection

_____ (c) the chemical processes of living organisms

Epidemiological studies may focus on isolating a carrier, which is usually difficult. But it is no easier to diagnose a hepatosplenic dysfunction.

a carrier carries
pathogenic organisms
but shows no symp-
toms of the disease

43: Why is it usually difficult to isolate a carrier? _____
_____
_____
_____

44: The dysfunction referred to involves (check one)

_____ (a) the heart and spleen

_____ (b) the intestine and liver

(c) the liver and spleen

_____ (c) the liver and spleen

_____ (d) the lip and lower jaw

45: Which word in the passage means "a bad or difficult
action of a body part"? _____

dysfunction

epi/demi/o

46: What word part means "upon the people"? _____/_____/_____

47: What word in the passage means "know completely"?

diagnose

_____

You have completed Unit 10. Look over your work carefully. You may work through the entire unit again, if you feel you need to do so.

R E V I E W   L I S T

This list of words is for your personal review. The number beside each word indicates the question in Unit 10 in which you began learning that word or word part. Space is provided for you to make notes for review.

physi/o (2)   **sub-** (19)

psych/o (4)   **hypo-** (22)

my/o (7)   **ex-** (23)

myc/o (10)   **dys-** (26)

myel/o (14)   **trans-** (30)

cutaneous (19)

Review Test for
Units 9 & 10

Directions: This review test covers the words and word parts learned in Units 9 and 10. *This is NOT a test to be graded.* It is for your use only. This is the final review test in the program. Before you elect to take your Final Test, you may want to review all five review tests. Make every effort to complete this review test; then check your answers with the answers on page 80.

1: An excision of the uvula is called a _____

Cocci that grow in a chain-like formation are _____

2: An infection within the ear may produce a draining of the ear. The general term meaning "a draining or discharge from the ear" is _____ .

3: Build a word that means "one who studies the ear, nose, and throat."

_____ / _____ / _____ / _____ / _____ / _____

4: Heart action is measured by a _____ .

Heart action is recorded by a _____ .

5: The recording produced by the second instrument named in 4 is called a _____ .

The process or science of making that recording is called _____ .

6: A patient who has lost a tooth through accident or disease may be fitted with an artificial tooth, called a _____ .

7: Mental functions are produced and developed in a process that is generally called

_____ / _____ / _____ .

8: A myelocyte is a cell in either the _____ or the

_____ .

9: Define mycophylaxin. _____

10: A myoneural mycopathy is a _____

_____ .

11: A subcutaneous mycosis occurs where? _____

_____ .

12: If a patient's arm forms a straight line between the shoulder and the wrist, the arm is

in an _____ position.

13: Define dysodontogenesis. _____

_____

14: To describe the action of an agent that passes through ("across") unbroken skin, you

could use either of two words: _____ or

_____ .

You have completed the review test for Units 9 and 10. Go over your work until you are satisfied that you have done your best. Then check your answers against the answers below. If you have any incorrect answers on this test, correct them at once. But leave a mark by those items which you missed, so that you may refer to them again in the future.

ANSWERS: UNITS 9 & 10

1. staphylectomy; streptococci
2. otorrhea
3. ot/o/rhin/o/laryng/o/log/ist
4. cardiometer; cardiograph
5. cardiogram; cardiography
6. dental prosthesis
7. psych/o/genesis
8. spinal cord; bone marrow
9. a preventative against fungus
10. a fungus-caused disease affecting both nerves and muscles
11. in the tissue below the skin
12. extended
13. bad or incorrect formation of the teeth
14. transdermic or transcutaneous

Section Two

Using The Health Sciences Library

Introduction

TO THE STUDENT:

This is the second section of *Terminology and Communication Skills in Health Sciences.* It consists of two self-instructional units on the resources and methods involved in using the health sciences library.

This section differs in some ways from Section One. You will be using both printed text and accompanying illustrations. You should read the directions carefully. You will be presented with *input, practice,* and *feedback,* just as you were in the terminology units.

But the learning responsibility is still on your shoulders. If you use this program honestly and conscientiously, you will learn what research resources are available in the typical health sciences library and how to locate them quickly.

OBJECTIVES:

1: You will be able to read correctly an entry in the card catalog or in the periodical index.

2: You will be able to locate a specific book or periodical article in the correct volume on the library shelf.

COMPONENTS:

This program consists of the following:

1: Two self-instructional Units.

2: Two Review Tests.

Every student in the health sciences must have a good working familiarity with the professional library. This program is designed to give you certain skills that will make your research easier and more effective. Work well, work at your own pace, and enjoy yourself.

Pre-Test:
Library Unit 1

Directions: This pre-test is designed to measure the knowledge that you presently have about the resources and research methods of the health sciences library. Answer as many of the questions as you can. Then check your answers with the correct answers on the next page. Please *do not* change any of your answers after turning the page.

1: A card in the health sciences library card catalog will tell you many things about a book. List three: **a)** _____ **b)** _____
   c) _____

2: Books and bound periodicals are listed in the card catalog by three means of identification. What are they? **a)** _____
   b) _____ **c)** _____

3: In the blanks provided, identify the elements of this entry from a periodical index.
   A dental fistula of unusual origin. Salman L.
New York J Dent 38:168-70, May 68

   a) author's name _____ **d)** page numbers _____
   b) volume number _____ **e)** periodical name _____
   c) issue date _____

4: Identify the elements of this entry in the blanks provided.
   12(5) : 41-52. 1966.

   a) first page of article _____ **c)** issue number _____
   b) volume number _____

5: List any three periodical indexes that you should find in the health sciences library.
   a) _____ **b)** _____
   c) _____

PRE-TEST ANSWERS

In Question 1, you could have listed title, author, city, date of publication, name of publisher, author's lifespan, number of pages, cross references, shelf location, and so on. In Question 2, you should have listed title, author, and subject, in any order. Question 3 should read like this: (a) Salman L.; (b) 38; (c) May 68; (d) 168-70; (e) New York J Dent. Question 4 should read like this: (a) 41; (b) 12; (c) 5. In Question 5, you could have listed *Index Medicus*, *Excerpta Medica*, *Index to Dental Literature*, *International Nursing Index*, *Biological Abstracts*, or others.

If your answers are 100 percent correct, skip to Unit 2.
If less than 100 percent correct, proceed with Unit 1.

UNIT 1

Directions: As you work through the unit, you should turn to the illustrations *only* when the directions tell you to do so. Remember it is very important that you do not look ahead in this book. You may *always* look back over your work, but you should *not* look ahead.

LIBRARY INDEXES:
  THE CARD CATALOG
  BOUND PERIODICAL INDEXES
  SPECIAL INDEXES (see UNIT 2)

In many respects, the health sciences library is similar to the arts and sciences library that you have often used. First, the health sciences library contains several *indexes*, which are nothing more than lists of the books, articles, and other materials that the library owns. Unit 1 will focus on the three categories of indexes: the *card catalog*, the *bound periodical indexes*, and the *special indexes*.

Generally, all indexes are alphabetized. Books and articles are listed by title, author, and subject in most library indexes. Any given book, for example, should be listed in at least three places in the index: it should be listed by its title, by the name of its author, and under the appropriate subject heading.

You'll find life among the indexes a lot easier if you can always look for a book by its title, because there is usually only one book with a given title. Unfortunately, it is often not that easy. If you know the author's name, you'll have to look a little harder, because the author may have written several books. Looking for a book by subject is the most difficult, because there may be 100 books under the same general subject heading.

1: Indexes are valuable library research tools because they list the _____ that the library owns.

2: Books and articles are usually indexed (listed) by _____ , _____ , and _____ .

3:    Under which index listing would you expect to find the greatest number of books or articles listed, "Jones, Robert T." (author) or "Mumps" (subject)? _____ Why? _____

_____

NOW CHECK YOUR ANSWERS

In Question 1, you should have answered that library indexes list the books, articles, and other materials that the library owns. In Question 2, you probably remembered that books and articles are usually indexed by author, title, and subject. In Question 3, you were correct if you wrote that the greatest number of books or articles would be listed under "Mumps," the subject heading. Common sense probably told you that while there may be hundreds of books written about "Mumps," Robert T. Jones probably has not published that many books all by himself.

THE CARD CATALOG:
The *card catalog* is a file that lists the shelf locations of all books and bound volumes of periodicals in the library. All volumes, both books and bound periodicals, that are on the library's shelves are listed on individual cards in the card catalog. When you are searching for a specific book or a specific volume of a bound periodical, check the card catalog to learn (1) *if* the library owns the volume, and (2) *where* on the shelves that volume is located.

4:    The card catalog lists the _____ of all books and bound periodical volumes in the library.

5:    The card catalog can give you two very useful pieces of information. What are they?

_____

_____

6:    You can waste a lot of time looking for an article that the library does not have. Once you know which bound volume the article is in, check the _____ to see if the library owns that specific volume.

NOW CHECK YOUR ANSWERS

In Question 4, you should have noted that the card catalog lists the shelf locations of all volumes, books, and bound periodicals in the library. In Question 5, you should have listed *if* the library owns the volume and *where* on the shelves the volume is located. In

Question 6, you should have answered that the card catalog is the place to check to be sure that the library owns the specific volume you're looking for. Makes sense, doesn't it?

Remember to fill in every blank in each question before looking ahead to check your answer.

There are two sections in the card catalog. One contains a list of volumes alphabetized by *subject*. In this section, books about "Hematology" will be listed before books about "Social Medicine." "Mental Health" will be listed before "Nursing Education."

7: The card catalog is divided into two sections, one of which lists books alphabetically by _____ .

8: Use numbers in the blanks to indicate the order in which the following would be listed in the subject section of the card catalog.

Pathology_____   a book titled *The Life of Tom Dooley* _____

Orthodontics _____   Public Health Administration _____

NOW CHECK YOUR ANSWERS

You should have named the subject section in Question 7. In Question 8, you probably numbered Orthodontics 1, Pathology 2, and Public Health Administration 3. You probably noticed that I tried to confuse you with a book *title*, which would not appear in the subject section at all.

The second section of the card catalog lists volumes *alphabetically by title* or *by author's name*. If you know the name of a given book's author—let's say Dr. John Smith—you can locate all the books by Dr. Smith *that the library owns* by checking the author/title section of the card catalog under "Smith, John." And if you know the title of the book—let's say *The Beat Goes on: A Study of the Heart*—you will find it listed under B (for *Beat*) in the author/title section. Remember, titles and authors are alphabetically/listed together in this section, so "Smith" would be listed after *Beat*.

9: The two sections of the card catalog are _____ and _____/_____ .

10: Which of the following would you *not* expect to find in the author/title section of the card catalog? _____

My Twenty Years Under Anesthetic
five books by Leon Christopher
a biochemistry professor
The Pre-Natal Clinic in the Urban Ghetto

11: Use numbers to indicate the order in which you would expect to find the following items listed in the author/title section of the card catalog.

George F. Meyers _____   *Cardiac Research Techniques* _____

The Brain _____   two books by Lucas Masters _____

12: How many cards listing *Problems in Radiology*, by Hugh Lewis, would you expect to find in the author/title section? _____

NOW CHECK YOUR ANSWERS

In Question 9, you should have named subject and author/title as the two sections of the card catalog. All the resources listed in Question 10 should be found in the author/title section—except for the biochemistry professor. For Question 11, you were right if you listed *The Brain* as 1, *Cardiac Research Techniques* 2, Lucas Masters 3, and George F. Meyers 4. You will always use this alphabetical approach to locating authors and titles in the card catalog. In Question 12, you should have said that two cards—one for the book's title and a separate one for the author's name—will list the book mentioned.

FIGURE 1

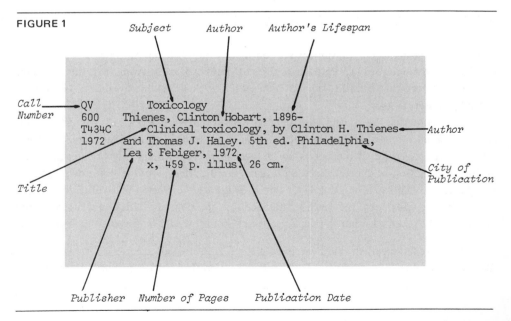

Figure 1 shows a typical card from the subject section of the card catalog. Look closely at the positions of the important pieces of information printed on this subject card.

a) Because it is a subject card, the subject heading—Toxicology—appears at the very top. In the average health sciences library, there are many cards under the general subject Toxicology.

b)   Next is the author's name: Thienes, Clinton Hobart. Further down on the card, you'll find that the book was written by both Thienes and Thomas J. Haley.

c)   The dates following the author's name indicate his lifespan. Thienes was born in 1896; there is no second date, so he is still living.

d)   The title of this book is *Clinical Toxicology*, and the library has the 5th edition.

e)   Philadelphia is the city where the book was published. The publishing company is Lea & Febiger. This edition of the book was published in 1972. You should always note the date of publication, because you will usually want only the latest published information in a health sciences field.

f)   The book's call number appears in the upper-left corner of the card. The number identifies the book's shelf location in the library. You'll learn more about using the call number, so remember what it looks like.

Examine Figure 1 closely to be sure you can recognize all the information that's printed on this card.

FIGURE 2

```
WL              Central nervous system - chemistry

300     McIlwain, Henry
M152          Biochemistry and the central nervous
1971    system, by Henry McIlwain and H.C. Bachelard.
        4th ed.  Edinburgh, Churchill Livingston,
        1971.
              vii, 616 p. illus. 24 cm.
```

The next few practice questions are based on the card catalog card that is shown in Figure 2.

13: From what section of the card catalog is this card taken? _____
     How do you know? _____

14: What is the title of this book? _____

15: Write the following information from the card: date of publication _____ ;
     city of publication _____ ; author's name _____

16: The card reproduced in Figure 1 was filed under the subject "Toxicology." Would the card in Figure 2 be filed in the card catalog before or after the "Toxicology" card? _____

NOW CHECK YOUR ANSWERS

If you looked carefully at this card, you recognized that it is taken from the subject section of the card catalog. As you should have answered in Question 13, the subject heading "Central nervous system—chemistry" appears at the top of the card. The title of the book, for Question 14, is *Biochemistry and the Central Nervous System*. In Question 15, you should have noted from the card that the book's date of publication is 1971, the city of publication is Edinburgh, and the author's name is Henry McIlwain (or McIlwain, Henry). "Central" is the first word in this card's subject heading. So it is filed before the "Toxicology" card—as you probably noted in Question 16.

FIGURE 3

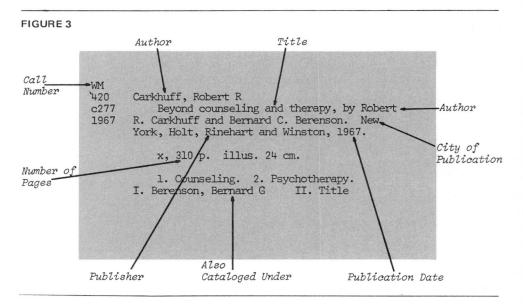

Figure 3 is a card from the author/title section of the card catalog. This, in fact, is an author card, which you recognize by seeing the author's name—"Carkhuff, Robert R."—at the top of the card. There is no subject heading on this card. This author card contains most of the vital information that you studied on the subject card. Take a look at it, and notice the locations of the following:

   a)   The author's name is followed by the title of the book, *Beyond Counseling and*

Therapy, which is followed by both authors' names: Carkhuff and Berenson. Whenever a book is coauthored, only one author's name appears at the top of the author card at a time; this is for purposes of alphabetizing.

b) The rest of the information on this card is presented in much the same way as information was presented on the subject card. Note the

> city and date of publication
> name of the publishing company
> number of pages in the book (310 pp.)

c) At the bottom of this card, you see the cross references, a list of the other headings under which this book is listed in the card catalog. You will find cards for this book under the subject heading "Counseling"; the subject heading "Psychotherapy"; the name of the coauthor, "Berenson, Bernard C."; and under the title of the book.

Examine this card very carefully before going on to the next illustration. Be sure that you can recognize all the important information that appears on the author card.

FIGURE 4

```
QV          Haley, Thomas J.
600      Thienes, Clinton Hobart, 1896-
T434c        Clinical toxicology, by Clinton H. Thienes
1972     and Thomas J. Haley.  5th ed. Philadelphia,
         Lea & Febiger, 1972
             x, 459 p. illus.  26 cm.
```

Look carefully at Figure 4 and answer the following questions:

17: Who wrote the book identified by this card? _____

18: You may also find this book listed under other headings. Name two with specific information from the card.

_____

_____

NOW CHECK YOUR ANSWERS

For Question 17, you should have listed both coauthors: Thomas J. Haley and Clinton Hobart Thienes. And in Question 18, you could have cited the book's title, the name of coauthor Thienes, or a subject heading such as "Toxicology."

When you are trying to find out if the library owns bound volumes of a given periodical—let's say the *Journal of the American Medical Association*—and where those volumes are located on the library shelves, check the author/title section of the card catalog. In the card catalog, the names of periodicals are treated like the titles of books. So, the *Journal of the American Medical Association* (*JAMA* for short) is the title of that periodical and is listed in the author/title section. You will also find periodicals listed in the subject section of the catalog, along with books. But to determine *if* the library owns bound volumes of a given periodical, *which* volumes the library owns, and *where* those volumes are shelved, you would be smart to check the author/title section first for the name of the periodical.

FIGURE 5

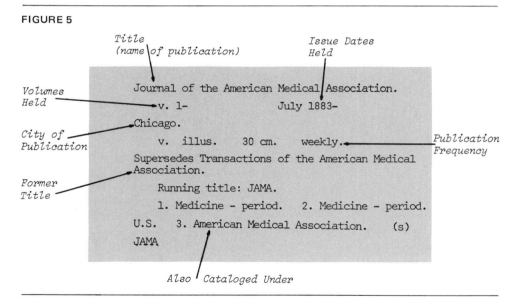

Figure 5 is a periodical card taken from the author/title section of the catalog. As you see, the "title" is *Journal of the American Medical Assocation*. Note the other important information that appears on this card.

   a)   The volumes of this periodical that the library owns are listed beneath the title.

In this case, the library holds all volumes from volume 1 to the present. (v.1⁻). If the library owned only some of the published volumes of the periodical, the card would indicate in this space which volumes the library owned.

b) A volume of a periodical is made up of several issues. So that you will know whether or not the library owns all the *issues* in all the *volumes*, this card also lists the issues that the library owns. In this case, the library owns all issues since the issue of July 1883.

c) Sometimes periodicals change their titles, so the periodical card may also note "former title," as this card does.

d) The entry "publication frequency" tells you how often this periodical is published. *JAMA* is published weekly.

e) Lower on the card you see a cross-reference list, which tells you the other headings under which this periodical is filed.

FIGURE 6

```
Bulletin of the Sloane Hospital for Women.
    v. 1-16; March 1955-Winter 1970.
New York, Sloane Hospital for Women.
    16 v. illus. 25 cm. quarterly.

    Full-title: Bulletin of the Sloane Hospital
for Women in the Columbia-Presbyterian Medical
Center, New York City.
    Continued as Sloane Hospital for Women journal.

    1. Gynecology - period.  2. Medicine - period.
-U.S.  3. Obstetrics - period.  I. Columbia-
Presbyterian Medical Center.   II. Sloane

Hospital for Women.
```

Figure 6 is a periodical card that contains all the information which you learned to recognize in Figure 5—and a little extra information, too. Look at Figure 6 carefully; then answer the following questions.

19: This card is taken from the author/title section of the card catalog. Would you expect to find it filed before or after the card for *JAMA*? _____
Would you expect to find it filed before or after the card for a periodical called the *Bulletin of Biological Research*? _____

20: How many volumes of this periodical does the library own? _____

21: Refer to two pieces of information on this card, and then do some mathematical calculations to answer this question. What is the total number of issues that the library owns? _____What two pieces of information did you use?

_____

_____

22: If you are looking for an article that is in volume 17 of this periodical, will you find it in this library? _____ How do you know? _____

_____

NOW CHECK YOUR ANSWERS

You probably wrote in Question 19 that you would find this card filed before the *JAMA* card. It would be filed after the *Biological Research* card, however, because when the first words in the titles are the same, you look to the second important words to find the alphabetical order. You should have looked at the "volumes held" note on the card and answered Question 20 with the number "16." To answer Question 21, you had to note that the library holds 15 years of issues and that four issues are published every year (publication frequency "quarterly"). Multiplication should have given you 60 issues as an answer. In Question 22, you should have answered "no," because the card tells you that the library owns volumes 1–16 only.

FIGURE 7

```
WL          Brain - Chemistry
300  McIlwain, Henry
M152        Biochemistry and the central nervous
1971 system, by Henry McIlwain and H.C. Bachelard.
        4th ed.  Edinburgh, Churchill Livingstone,
        1971.
            vii, 616 p.  illus. 24 cm.
            Includes bibliography.
```

Now look carefully at Figure 7; then answer the following review questions.

23: Under what heading is this card filed? _____

In what section of the card catalog? _____

24: In the space to the right, write in the call number from this card. _____

FIGURE 8

```
        Medicine - periodicals
   Journal of the American Medical Association.
        v. 1-            July 1883-
   Chicago.
        v.  illus.  30 cm.  weekly.

   For further information see main entry card.
```

25: How many pages are in this book? _____

26: Look carefully at Figure 8. Is the card referring to a book, an audiovisual program, a periodical, or some other material? _____

27: How many volumes does the library own? Check one.

one volume _____   volumes 1-10 _____

no volumes _____   all volumes to date _____

NOW CHECK YOUR ANSWERS

In Figure 7, you were looking at a card from the subject section of the card catalog, as you should have noted in answering Question 23. The card would be filed under "Brain—chemistry." The card number you wrote for Question 24 appeared in the upper-left corner of the card; it began with a WL and ended with the date 1971. Does that look familiar? For Question 25, you should have answered 616 pages. The answer to Question 26, as you observed in Figure 8, is "periodical." And because the card in Figure 8 indicates "1-", you should have checked "all volumes to date" in Question 27.

If you were able to identify most of the information requested in review questions 23-27, you're doing very well in this unit. Keep up the good work!

BOUND PERIODICAL INDEXES:

The *bound periodical indexes* in the health sciences library are similar in many ways to the *Readers' Guide to Periodical Literature*, which you have used in high school and college. The periodical indexes are sets of volumes that alphabetically list the articles and reports published in professional journals, magazines, and other periodicals. These idexes can direct you to

1. the specific periodical
2. the correct volume
3. the correct issue
4. the exact page

where a given article is published.

Major periodical indexes include: *Index Medicus*, *Excerpta Medica*, *Biological Abstracts*, *Index to Dental Literature*, and *International Nursing Index*. They are all for both general and specialty use. But this is only representative; there are many other indexes that you may need to use during your health sciences education.

Nearly all periodical indexes share the following characteristics:

a) They list articles and reports published in journals, magazines, and other periodicals.

b) Most indexes list articles by subject and author. A few indexes also list by title.

c) Periodical indexes list articles from a great number of periodicals. A few list foreign as well as U.S. publications.

d) You probably won't find articles less than 4 months old listed in the periodical indexes. Articles less than 4 months old can probably be located on the "current periodicals" shelves of the library.

e) An entry in a periodical index will give you a lot of important information: an article's title and author, the periodical name, volume, issue date, and page numbers. But the entry will *not* tell you if the library owns that volume of the periodical. You must check the card catalog for that information.

The *Index Medicus* (*IM*) and the *Quarterly Cumulative Index Medicus* (*QCIM*) make up one of the major professional periodical indexes in the health sciences library. You may consider the *IM* and the *QCIM* as one index made up of many volumes, arranged by years (chronologically). The *IM* lists articles by subject and by author.

28: Both the card catalog and the periodical indexes are useful in locating articles and reports published in professional periodicals. The major difference between them is that the card catalog lists _____ and the periodical index lists _____ .

29: You should not expect to find an article less than _____ listed in a periodical index. Look for recent articles on the _____ shelves.

30: The *Index Medicus* is divided into volumes by _____ . It lists articles both by _____ and by _____ .

31: Which of the following items of information should you *not* expect to find in a periodical index?

      a) article titles _____   **c)** authors' names _____

      b) periodical volume numbers_____   **d)** volume shelf locations _____

NOW CHECK YOUR ANSWERS

In Question 28, you probably answered that the card catalog lists the shelf locations of volumes and the periodical index lists individual articles and authors. You should have remembered for Question 29 that an article less than 4 months old is not likely to be listed in a periodical index. In Question 30, you should have written that *IM* is divided into volumes by years, and that it lists articles by author and by subject. For Question 30, you only had to check item (d).

FIGURE 9

```
MYELOGRAPHY (E1)

Value of Myelography in thoracic spinal cord injuries.
   Cantu RC.  Int Surg 56: 23-6, Jul 71

Smitherman TC, Moss HM, Riesz P: Radiation-induced
   hydrogen transfer in nucleic acids, proteins, and
   related substances;  effects of temperature and
   scavengers.  Radiat Res 46:251-67, May 71
```

Now that you have a lot of good information about the general nature of periodical indexes, let's look at some individual entries in *IM*. Figure 9 shows both a subject entry and an author entry. Look first at the subject entry and note the following items of information:

    a)   The major subject heading, "MYELOGRAPHY," is printed in bold type, and it is in alphabetical order in the subject section.

    b)   The title of the article, "Value of myelography," is on the first line of the entry.

    c)   The author's name, Cantu RC, follows the title.

d) Next, in bold type, is the name of the periodical in which the article is published. The periodical names are usually abbreviated. This one means *Internal Surgery*.

e) The first number in the series of numbers following the name of the periodical is the volume number in which the article appears, in this case, volume 56.

f) Following the volume number and the colon (:) are the page numbers on which the article appears.

g) The last item in the entry is the date (July 1971) of the issue in which the article appears.

Put them all together and you have enough information to help you find the periodical, volume, issue, and page where the article you're looking for is published. Of course, you do need to check the card catalog, too.

Now look again at the author entry in Figure 9. As you see, the name of the author or authors is in bold type. The title of the article or report follows the author's name, and it's normal type. Then comes the name of the periodical, the volume and page numbers, and the issue date. Both subject and author entries contain much the same information; it's just arranged a little differently.

32: Look closely at the author entry in Figure 9. What are the names of the authors of this article (as they appear in the entry)? _____

33: What is the abbreviated name of the periodical in which the Smitherman article is published? _____

34: Look once again at the author entry and fill in these blanks:
volume number _____   page number(s)_____
issue date _____

NOW CHECK YOUR ANSWERS

In Question 32, you naturally answered Smitherman TC, Moss HM, and Riesz P. In Question 33, you wrote the abbreviation Radiat Res (which stands for *Radiation Research*, as you probably guessed). For 34, you only needed to note that the volume number is 46, the page numbers are 251–67, and the issue date is May 71.
Here are a few more practice questions, based on the index entries that you see in Figure 10.

35: Who is the author of the article referred to in the subject entry? _____

36: Complete the following blanks with information from the author entry:
    a) page numbers _____   **b)** issue date _____
    c) abbreviated periodical name _____

FIGURE 10

ETIOLOGY

Pathogenesis of cutaneous Marek's disease in chickens.
    Lapen RF, et al.   J Natl Cancer Inst 47:389-99
    Aug 71

Frankenfeld FM, Black HJ, Dick RW: Automated
    formulary printing from a computerized drug
    information file. Am J Hosp Pharm 28:155-61,
    Mar 71

37: In what volume of the *Journal of the National Cancer Institute* will you find an article about the development of a skin disease in chickens? _____
In what issue? _____

38: If both of these entries were in the author section of *IM*, which would be filed first?

_____

39: After you have noted all the information from the entry on the article by Lapen, what would be your next two steps in the process of locating the article? Step 1

_____

Step 2 _____

NOW CHECK YOUR ANSWERS

For Question 35, you identified the article titled "Pathogensis of . . ." as the subject entry and found that the author is Lapen RF. Then you should have completed the blanks in Question 36 as follows: (a) 155–61; (b) Mar(ch) 71; (c) Am J Hosp Pharm. Question 37 referred to the subject entry, of course, in which you found the article in volume 47, issue date Aug(ust) 71. You probably did the correct thinking for Question 38 and decided that since "F" comes before "L," the Frankenfeld article would be listed first in the author section. Question 39 called on you to remember that you should go *first* to the card catalog to find the periodical's shelf location, and *second* to the shelf to find the correct volume.

We will now look at the forms of a few other major periodical index entries. You'll find that much of the same information appears in all of them, but in somewhat different forms. You have probably learned a lot about reading an *Index Medicus* entry, and you'll be learning a lot about other indexes, too.

FIGURE 11

```
    12.  ABNORMALITIES OF THE SYSTEMIC CIRCULATION

         a.   ESSENTIAL ARTERIAL HYPERTENSION, MALIGNANT
              HYPERTENSION, NEPHROGENIC HYPERTENSION

   105.  THE CHANGING OUTLOOK FOR THE HYPERTENSIVE PATIENT
         Page J.H. Res. Div. Cleveland Clin. Found.,
         Cleveland O. - ANN. INTER. MED. 1962, 57/1
         (96-109) Graphs 1 Tables 2 illus. 2.
```

Another major periodical index in the health sciences library is the *Excerpta Medica (EM)*. This index is also a large set of volumes divided chronologically. But the *EM* is also divided by medical specialty, and each medical specialty group is divided chronologically. When you look at a set of *EM* on the library shelf, you will see the Cardiology section consisting of several volumes arranged chronologically. The Hematology section is also arranged chronologically, and so on through the entire *EM*.

As you look at Figure 11, you see that the information in this typical *EM* entry is much like the information that you have learned to recognize in *Index Medicus* entries. But there are a few differences. Look closely at the arrangement of the following bits of information on this *EM* entry:

   a) The subject heading, "Abnormalities of the Systematic Circulation," appears in bold type.
   b) The information beneath the subject heading is a list of the subject subareas that are covered by articles filed under this heading.
   c) Next is a sample entry, with the title of the article in bold type.
   d) The author is identified in *EM* entries by name and by institution; in this entry the author, Page J.H., is with the Research Division of the Cleveland Clinical Foundation.

e) The name of the periodical in which this article is published is abbreviated in bold type, followed by the volume number 57, and an issue number 1 instead of an issue date.

f) In parentheses you see the page numbers in issue 1 of volume 57 where you will find Page's article.

g) The next items of information in this entry inform you that the article includes 1 graph, 2 tables, and 2 illustrations.

In the *Excerpta Medica*, each entry like the one you have just looked at is followed by an abstract, or brief description, of the contents of the article. The abstract is very handy.

Look over Figure 11 again, until you are sure that you recognize all the important information in this *EM* entry.

FIGURE 12

```
108.  HEMOSYNAMIC ALTERATIONS ACCOMPANYING DIASTOLIC
      HYPERTENSION - Novack D. Cardiovasc. Sec. Dept.
      of Med. Hahnemann Med. Coll. and Hosp.
      Philadelphia, Pa. - AMER. J. CARDIOL., 1962
      9/5 (659-662)

Essential hypertension is generally characterized by a
normal cardiac output with increased peripheral resis-
tance due to a reduction in the cross-section area of
the arterial vascular bed.  The consequence of such
hypertension on the hemodynamic changes in the brain,
kidneys and heart are reviewed. (XVIII, 6*)
```

Look carefully at the *EM* entry in Figure 12. The next few questions are based on this illustration.

40: In what year was this article published? _____ In what periodical (use abbreviation)? _____

41: Identify the meanings of 9/5 _____ and (659–662) _____

42: Who is the article's author? _____

Good! Now check the following feedback to see how well you did on those practice questions.

NOW CHECK YOUR ANSWERS

A quick glance at the entry helped you answer 1962 as the year of publication for Question 40, and for the name of the periodical you wrote AMER. J. CARDIOL. For Question 41, you probably said that 9 is the volume number, 5 the issue number, and 659–662 the page numbers on which the article appears. And for Question 42, it was easy to identify Novack D. (or D. Novack) as the author.

FIGURE 13

A   882289, WILLIAMS T. FRANKLIN. EVELYN ANDERSON. JULIA D. WATKINS and VIRGINIA COYLE. (Dep. Prev. Med. Univ. N.C., Chapel Hill, N.C. U.S.A.) Dietary errors made at home by patients with diabetes. J. AMER. DIET. ASS. 51 (1): 19-25 Illus. 1967 – a sample was drawn from medically indigent diabetic patients attending 2 univ-

   MORTALITY
B   Acute coronary care – a five year report. Day H.W. Amer. Cardiol. 21: 252-7, Feb 68

   OSTEOTOMY
C   Oral surgery for the correction of facial skeletal deformities White RP Jr. et al. J. Kentucky Dent. Ass. 20: 9-15 Jan 68

In Figure 13, you see sample entries from four more periodical indexes. Remember that there are many indexes available to you in the health sciences library. This unit is dealing with the most representative ones. Learn to read these entries accurately and you'll be able to read nearly all of them.

Sample A is from *Biological Abstracts*, an index to articles, published in English and foreign-language periodicals, that deal in some way with the biological aspects of health science. Note that the principal division of *Biological Abstracts* is by years. But it is also divided by subject. In this individual entry, the identification number is followed by the names of the authors in bold type. Then follow (1) the name of the institution where the research for the article was done; (2) the title, in lower case type and underlined; (3) the name of the periodical; (4) the volume number and then the issue number in parentheses; (5) the page numbers where the article appears. A note that the article is illustrated and the year of publication are followed by an abstract, or summary, of the article's contents. That seems like a lot of information, but it all makes sense. Take another look at it.

43: The index called *Biological Abstracts* lists articles that deal with the _____ aspects of health science.

44: In what volume of the periodical does this article appear? _____
What issue number? _____ What year? _____

Sample B is from the *International Nursing Index* for 1968. The entry you see here is listed under "Coronary Disease." The first line in this entry contains the title of the article, followed by the name of the author. The name of the periodical is abbreviated in bold type. Then follow (1) the volume number of the periodical, (2) the page numbers in the specific issue, and (3) the date of that issue. Pretty clear and straightforward, don't you think?

45: Look at Sample B. What is the title of the article? _____
_____ .

46: What is the issue date in Sample B? _____

Sample C in Figure 13 is taken from the *Index to Dental Literature*. The first entry under the subject heading "Osteotomy" refers to an article published in the *Journal of the Kentucky Dental Association*. Look at it very carefully. Then using what you have learned about reading entries in professional periodical indexes, answer the following questions.

47: Assume that you are standing before the library shelf containing bound volumes of the *Journal of the Kentucky Dental Association*. Which volume will you select if you want to read the article referred to in Sample C? _____

48: You have the volume in your hand. You should now flip through the volume until you reach the issue for _____ .

49: You are looking at the first page of the issue identified in Question 48. What page will you turn to? _____

NOW CHECK YOUR ANSWERS

Now let's take a few minutes to check your work in questions 43-49. In Question 43, you probably filled the blank with the word "biological." In Question 44, you should have listed volume 51, issue number 1, and the year 1967. Then in Question 45, you should have answered that the title of the article in Sample B is "Acute coronary care—a five year report." The issue date in Sample B (Question 46) is Feb(ruary) 68. In Question 47, you started by selecting volume 20. In Question 48 you turned to the issue for January 1968. And in Question 49 you began reading on page 9.

Here's a chance to get in a little more practice reading periodical index entries before you take the review test for this unit. There are four entries or parts of entries in Figure 14. Look at them carefully, then answer the following practice questions.

FIGURE 14

```
A    73:  177-178, MAY 20 '70

B    62/5   (24-32)

C    110(65): 290-292   1954

D    Acute coronary care.  Day H.W.
     Amer J Cardiol 21: 252-7    Feb 68
```

50: In Sample A, what is the volume number of the periodical? _____

51: In Sample B, what does 62/5 mean? 62 is the _____ ;
5 is the _____ .

52: In Sample C, should you look for an issue date or an issue number? _____
What is that date or number? _____

53: Look at Samples A, C, and D. Which of the articles referred to was published first?
_____ Which was published next? _____

NOW CHECK YOUR ANSWERS

In Question 50, the volume number is 73. In Question 51, you probably noted that 62 is the periodical volume number and 5 the issue number. For Question 52, you wrote that Sample C contains an issue number, which is number 65. And in Question 53, you should have found that Sample C refers to the year 1954, which is earliest, and that Sample D includes the issue date "Feb 68," which is next. From the information given, there's no way to know the publication date for Sample B.

You have completed Unit 1. Please check your work to be sure that you have answered as many of the practice questions as possible.

Review Test for Unit 1

1: Among the useful research tools in the health sciences library are the indexes, which for the purposes of this unit, fall into three general types. What are they?

   a) _____ b) _____

   c) _____

2: The card catalog lists books by _____ , by _____ , and by _____ .

3: The card catalog also contains vital information about articles that can be found in the library. What are two of the most important pieces of information? (a) _____

   _____

   b) _____

   _____

4: Use numbers to indicate the order in which the following would be listed in the subject section of the card catalog.

   Microbiology _____   Biochemistry _____

   Osteomalacia _____   Passive Diffusion _____

5: Which of the following items of information would you *not* expect to find on a card catalog book card? (Indicate with checkmark.)

   city of publication_____   author's name _____

   number of copies sold _____   date of publication _____

6: What major periodical index would be most likely to list an article on nursing care for the elderly? _____

7: An article *less than 4 months old* will probably be located among the _____ .

8: Look carefully at the following fictional entry from a periodical index. Then fill in the blanks below.

A dental fistula of unusual origin. Salman L.
New York J Dent 38:168–70, May 68

   a) abbreviated name of periodical _____
   b) page numbers _____
   c) issue date _____
   d) volume number _____
   e) author's name _____

9: Which of the items of information that you listed in Question 8 will you need to locate this article in its bound volume? _____

10: Here's another fictional entry. Look at it carefully, then fill in the blanks below.

12(3) : 66–70. 1966.

   a) page number on which article begins _____
   b) issue number _____
   c) volume number _____

11: After you have noted the information in a periodical index entry, what further information do you need to locate the article? _____

12: List three major periodical indexes that you should find in any health sciences library.

   a) _____
   b) _____
   c) _____

You have completed the Library Review Test. Look over your work carefully. When you are satisfied that you have done your best on this test, check the answers below. If you have missed any answers, correct them at once. But leave a mark by those corrected so that you may locate them in the future.

ANSWERS: UNIT 1

1. a) card catalog
   b) periodical indexes
   c) special indexes

2. title, author, and subject

3. a) whether or not the library owns the necessary volume of the periodical
   b) where the volume is shelved

4. a) Biochemistry   c) Osteomalacia
   b) Microbiology   d) Passive Diffusion

5. number of copies sold

6. *International Nursing Index*

7. current periodicals

8. a)   New York J. Dent
   b)   168–70
   c)   May 68
   d)   38
   e)   Salman L.

9. all except (e), author's name

10. a)   66
    b)   3
    c)   12

11. card catalog information on whether or not library owns that volume and its location

12. You may list any three, including *Index Medicus, Excerpta Medica, Index to Dental Literature, Biological Abstracts, International Nursing Index*, or others.

Pre-Test: Library Unit 2

Directions: This pre-test is designed to measure your present knowledge of the material contained in Unit 2. Cover the bottom half of this page with a folded piece of paper. Answer as many of the questions as you can; then check your answers with the answers at the bottom of the page. Please *do not* change any of your answers after checking the correct answers.

1: On the lines provided, identify the meanings of each segment of the following library call number.

WR _____

413 _____

J12c _____

1951 _____

2: Is the book identified by the call number in Question 1 shelved in the main shelving section or the reference section? _____

How do you know? _____

3: Look at the following sample index entry. What page numbering system does this periodical use? _____

15 : 985–991 Je 38

4: List three health sciences library shelving sections other than the main section. (a) ___
_____ (b) _____

(c) _____

PRE-TEST ANSWERS

Your answers in Question 1 should read like this: WR, shelving section; 413, shelving subsection; the J in J12c, author's last initial; 1951, publication date. The book (Question 2) is in the main shelving section; there would be a "ref" or "reference" in the call number if it were in the reference section. You'd be safe in answering 3 with the term "consecutive numbering system." In 4, you could have listed the reference, government documents, and microfilm sections.

If your answers are *less* than 100 percent correct, proceed with Unit 2.

UNIT 2

Directions: Unit 2 is similar to Unit 1. The important thing to remember while you're working through this unit is not to look ahead. If you're going to learn as much as possible in this unit, please *do not* look ahead.

First, here's a quick review of several important things to remember from Unit 1:

* The card catalog lists all volumes in the health sciences library—both books and bound periodicals. If you can't find a book or periodical card in the card catalog, the library doesn't have that book or periodical.
* The card catalog lists the shelf locations of all volumes.
* The periodical indexes list articles published in professional journals. There are general indexes, such as *Index Medicus*, and special indexes, such as the *Index to Hospital Literature*.
* The general procedure for finding an article in a professional periodical follows these steps:
  * Locate the article in the periodical index, carefully noting all information from the index entry.
  * Find the volume's shelf location in the card catalog.
  * Find the article by page numbers in the volume.

Below is a sample call number, which would appear in the upper-left corner of a card catalog card. Look at it carefully.

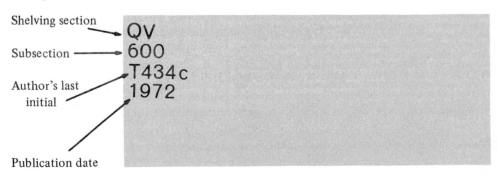

Shelving section → QV

Subsection → 600

Author's last initial → T434c

Publication date → 1972

This *call number* is based on the Dewey Decimal System of library cataloging, a fact that you need not remember as long as you can use the call number efficiently. Study the four important items of information contained in this call number:

* The first two letters indicate the area among the book stacks where this book is shelved. The QV shelving section should be easy to find, since shelving sections are arranged alphabetically.

* The number on the second line indicates the shelving subsection where this book may be found. When you have located the QV shelving section, it should be easy to find 600, since subsections are arranged in numerical order.

* The third line in the call number begins with the first initial of the author's last name. This is just another means of identifying this book among several that might be in the same section and subsection.

* The publication date does not appear in all call numbers. If the book you are seeking has been revised a few times, this date is helpful in finding the revision edition you're looking for.

Now look back at the call number sample. Study it carefully to prepare for a little practice with another call number.

Look closely at the following sample book call number and answer the few practice questions that follow.

WP
710
R4

1: Which of the pieces of information in the call number above would you use *first* in locating this book on the shelf? _____

2: Given the following selection, who is most likely to be the author of this book? Check one.

John J. Wright _____   Dr. Margaret Johnson _____

Hector Farias, Ph.D. ____   Dr. Carl Rogers _____

3: You might assume that this book has not been published in any other edition because there is no _____ in the call number

NOW CHECK YOUR ANSWERS

Well, that was a pretty easy set of practice questions, wasn't it? In Question 1, you had no trouble answering that the shelving section letters, WP, would be the first item of information you would use in locating this book. Since the letter "R" appears in the third line of the call number, it's most likely that Dr. Carl Rogers is the author in Question 2. And for Question 3, the fact that there is no publication date in the call number might lead you to assume that this book has not been published in an earlier edition.

Here are a couple of good points to remember. First, a call number is like an address. If you use it correctly, you should easily be able to locate any volume in the library, unless that volume has been checked out. Whenever you have an extraordinary amount of trouble locating a book on the shelf, ask for assistance from library personnel.

Second, even if you have the world's sharpest memory, you should always write down such information as the *complete* call number from a catalog card. You can get into a real mess if you forget just one letter or number of the call number. So apply this general rule when you're doing library research: always write it down!

Imagine that you have found an article listed in a periodical index and have jotted down all the important information from the index entry. You have checked the card catalog to be sure that the library owns that particular volume of that particular periodical. You are now standing in the library with the correct volume in your hand. Now what?

19: 39-43 Je 71

Referring to the information that you have noted from the index entry, you flip through volume 19 until you find the issue dated June 1971. Then, when you turn to page 39, you should be looking right at the article you need.

There is something else you should know about page numbers.

AMER.J.CARDIOL. 1962, 9/5 (663-668)

This entry is an example of a journal in which the pages are not numbered *issue by issue*, but *consecutively* through each volume. In an issue by issue numbering system, issue 1 in a given volume might contain pages 1-40; issue 2, pages 1-38; issue 3, pages 1-43; and so on. Each issue begins with page number 1 in the issue by issue numbering system.

But in the consecutive-page-numbering system, issue 1 contains pages 1-40; issue 2, pages 41-79; issue 3, pages 80-123; and so on. So in the AMER. J. CARDIOL., volume 9, issue 5 may contain pages 552-670. In this case, you only need to look through volume 9 for the page numbers of your article. You *don't* need to look for the issue.

4: There are two systems of page numbering in professional periodicals. What are they?
    a) _____   b) _____
5: When you are using a journal with the _____ numbering system, you only need to look for page numbers within the volume, not issue numbers or dates.

6: In the _____ numbering system, page 1 appears at the first of each issue. In the _____ system, page 1 appears at the first of each volume.

NOW CHECK YOUR ANSWERS.

In Question 4, you should have easily responded that the two page numbering systems are the issue-by-issue and consecutive numbering systems. You can get by with using page numbers only when the journal has a consecutive numbering system (Question 5). And you probably remembered in Question 6 that page 1 appears at the first of each issue in an issue-by-issue numbering system and at the first of each volume in a consecutive numbering system.

You encountered a lot of input when working Library Unit 1, and you probably mastered most of it. By the time you complete Unit 2 you will have a good working knowledge of the health sciences library and will be able to locate research materials without much difficulty. As in all things involving the learning of new skills, however, library research becomes easier as you gain more experience in it. So, keep up the good work!

In the first few pages of Unit 2, you have learned how to locate most volumes in the health sciences library. Now let's take a look at some of the exceptional systems by which libraries shelve books and periodicals.

If you have traced a volume to the place where it *should* be on the library shelf and you find that it's not there, you may locate it somewhere nearby. If a given volume is too large to fit the normal shelf space, for instance, it may be out of its call-number order—perhaps on the end of the shelf. Keep such a possibility in mind. If you can't immediately locate a volume, scout around a little. But *don't waste a lot of time looking for volumes that aren't where they should be*; ask for assistance.

In some libraries, volumes are shelved not by call numbers but by specialty. So you may find that all publications in the area of Public Health are shelved together, all Pharmacy publications may be shelved together, and so on. This practice is a little confusing at first; but when you have learned where these specialty areas are, it's more convenient for the researcher. At least, that's the theory.

Government documents and reports, such as federal studies on population planning, are usually shelved in a special area. Ask a librarian where the government documents are located. Sometimes government documents are even indexed in a separate card catalog.

If you find a catalog card that has the words "microfilm" or "micro" in or near the call number, you know that the book or periodical is stored in microfilm in the library.

Ask for directions to the microfilm shelving area, find the correct microfilm by call number, and read it with the help of the library's microfilm reading equipment.

7: If you have traced a volume to its correct shelf location and find that it's not there, what are three reasons that might explain the situation?   a) _____

_____

b) _____

_____ c) _____

_____

8: A professor has mentioned a government research project in an area that you're interested in. You can't find any mention of the project report in the major indexes. Where should you look? _____

_____

9: The notation "microfilm" on a catalog card should send you first to _____ _____, where you locate your volume by _____ . Then, to do your reading, you will have to use the library's _____ .

NOW CHECK YOUR ANSWERS

In Question 7, you could have listed a number of possibilities, but your best answers would include the volume's size being too big for the shelf, the volume being shelved in a specialty area, the volume being among government documents or on microfilm, or the volume being in use by another student. In Question 8, you probably answered that you would look in the government documents shelving area and, possibly, check a special documents index. And in Question 9, the word "microfilm" should send you to the microfilm shelving area, where you locate your volume by call number, and then to the microfilm reading equipment.

You have just learned a few things that some health sciences students don't learn for years. Consider yourself ahead of the game.

The reference section in the health sciences library is much like the reference section in an undergraduate arts and sciences library. It is a shelving area for volumes of specialized information, volumes that cannot be checked out of the library. The words "reference" or "ref" on a catalog card will send you to the reference section. There you can use the library's professional encyclopedias and dictionaries. The reference section also shelves volumes such as the professional *Who's Who* and other directories listing men and women in the health sciences, where they are working, and the nature of their professional interests. And the reference section shelves equipment catalogs, audiovisual aids, catalogs, and the like.

10: If the call number on a catalog card includes the notation "ref," you will find that volume in the _____ .

11: In a conversation with fellow students, you hear the name "Dr. Hugo Katzenklunk" several times. You don't confess that you never heard of Katzenklunk, and you want to find out about him. A good place to find the basic facts about Katzenklunk's education and professional interests is probably a book in _____ _____ .

12: If your laboratory director tells you that you must buy a microscope, you can find out what's available in such equipment by checking the _____ in the reference section.

N O W   C H E C K   Y O U R   A N S W E R S

In Question 10, you had a chance to show that "ref" in a call number will send you to the library's reference section. While you're in the reference section, you can look up Katzenklunk (Question 11) in a professional directory or *Who's Who*. Microscopes and other technical gear, such as you need in Question 12, can be found in equipment catalogs in the reference section.

You have completed Unit 2. Look over your work in this unit carefully.

Review Test for
Unit 2

Directions: This review test, like all review tests in this program, is *not* a test to be graded. It is for your use only, and it is designed to help you check your learning progress. Make an honest effort to complete each blank in each question of this review test. Then, when you have done your best, check your work with the answers on page 120.

1: Examine the sample call number below, then supply the information called for in the blanks.

AS
413
P8.2
1960

a) publication date ＿＿＿＿＿＿＿ c) shelving section ＿＿＿＿＿＿＿

b) subsection ＿＿＿＿＿＿＿ d) author's initial ＿＿＿＿＿＿＿

2: Is the book identified by the call number in Question 1 in the reference section or the main shelving area? ＿＿＿＿＿＿＿＿＿＿＿＿＿＿＿＿＿＿

How do you know? ＿＿＿＿＿＿＿＿＿＿＿＿＿＿＿＿＿＿

3: When you have located the correct volume, what further information must you use to locate a specific article? ＿＿＿＿＿＿＿＿＿＿＿＿＿＿＿＿

4: Take a look at the sample index entry below. What page numbering system does this periodical use? ＿＿＿＿＿＿＿＿＿＿＿＿＿＿＿＿＿＿

27: 1021–1050 Oct 68

5: What is the reason that you answered Question 4 as you did?

＿＿＿＿＿＿＿＿＿＿＿＿＿＿＿＿＿＿＿＿＿＿＿＿＿＿＿＿＿＿

＿＿＿＿＿＿＿＿＿＿＿＿＿＿＿＿＿＿＿＿＿＿＿＿＿＿＿＿＿＿

6: Along with the main shelving area, what are two other shelving areas that you should be familiar with? a) ＿＿＿＿＿＿＿＿＿＿＿＿＿＿＿＿

b) ＿＿＿＿＿＿＿＿＿＿＿＿＿＿＿＿

You have completed the Library Review Test for Unit 2. Check your work with the answers below. Correct any answers that you may have missed.

ANSWERS: UNIT 2

1. (a) 1960; (b) 413; (c) AS; (d) P;

2: Main shelving area, because there is no "reference" notation in the call number.

3: Sometimes the issue number or date, but always the page numbers.

4. It probably uses the consecutive numbering system.

5. The page numbers (1021–1050) are so high that it is likely that page 1 is at the first of the volume rather than at the first of the issue.

6. Government documents, specialty, reference (choose two)

Section Three

Organization and Expression for the Health Professional

Introduction

TO THE STUDENT:

This series of self-instructional units on organization and expression is designed to help strengthen your communication skills. The verbal skills taught in this program are those that you will use most often during your years as a health sciences student and as a practicing professional. You will learn things and practice skills that are directly relevant to your need for them. Nothing is taught in these units that does not have some practical application. There are no "rules for rules' sake" here. There are no literary exercises. What you see in these units is what you get, and what you get is what you need.

OBJECTIVES:
1: You will correctly identify a specified number of grammatical and syntactical errors in assigned reading.
2: You will write a series of correctly constructed sentences containing elements of topic, exposition, and conclusion.
3: You will write a correctly organized paragraph.
4: You will write a multiple-paragraph paper containing elements of topic, exposition, transition, and conclusion.

COMPONENTS:
This program contains the following:
1: Three self-instructional Units.
2: One Review Test.

Remember that the responsibility for using these units according to directions is still on your shoulders. Work carefully and work at your own pace.

Pre-Test:
Organization Unit 1

Directions: This pre-test is designed to measure your skills in organization and expression. To use this pre-test correctly, complete as much of the work on this page as you can. Then check your answers below. Please *do not* change any work on this page after checking the answers.

In the following sentences there are grammatical and structural errors. Underline the error in each sentence and rewrite the sentence correctly.

1: Megalomania is not an attribute of a good physician and can lead them to expect unattainable successes.

2: The patient, still dressed in his examining gown, run through the halls of the clinic.

3: To learn more of Doctor Smith's work and making use of his findings are responsibilities of the modern practitioner.

4: Pharmacy following the lead of private research laboratories and instituting programs of research into digitalis overdosage complications.

5: In completing her tasks, the dental assistant to sterilize all equipment.

6: Doctors must be aware of the limitations of his science and personal knowledge.

When you have checked your work carefully, compare it with the correct answers, which follow.

PRE-TEST ANSWERS

1. Underline them
   Megalomania is not an attribute of a good physican and can lead *him* to expect unattainable successes.

2. Underline run
   The patient, still dressed in his examining gown, *ran* (or *runs*) through the halls of the clinic.

3. Underline either <u>to learn</u> or <u>making</u>

   Learning more of Doctor Smith's work and making use of his findings are responsibilities of the modern practitioner.

   or

   To learn more of Doctor Smith's work and *to make* use of his findings are responsibilities of the modern practitioner.

4. Underline <u>following</u>

   Pharmacy *is following* the lead of private research laboratories and instituting programs of research into digitalis overdosage complications.

5. Underline <u>to sterilize</u>

   In completing her tasks, the dental assistant *sterilizes* (or *sterilized*) all equipment.

6. Underline <u>his</u>

   Doctors must be aware of the limitations of *their* science and personal knowledge.

If your work on this pre-test was 100 percent correct, skip to Pre-Test 2; if *less* than 100 percent correct, proceed to Unit 1.

UNIT 1

Let's begin by refreshing our memories. First, recall that every sentence needs both a *subject* and a *verb*. At least one of the sentences in the pre-test to this unit needed a verb. Of course, everybody knows this, but sometimes things get out of control and the verb gets left out or gets used in the wrong form. For instance:

> In each case, the infected carrier
> without being carefully sterilized
> according to hospital regulations.

This string of words makes sense, because the reader supplies by guesswork the words that have been left out. But if the reader isn't that generous, then communication fails. *If you're in the health sciences, you're in a profession that demands clarity of communication.* So

EVERY SENTENCE MUST HAVE
BOTH A <u>SUBJECT</u> AND A [VERB].

Locate the subject and the verb in each of the following sentences. Mark the subject by <u>underlining</u> it. Enclose the verb in [brackets].

1: Four instances of staphylococcus infection were reported by the nursing staff.
2: Becoming hysterical with fright, the child soon exhibited cyanoderma.
3: Three community health agencies have adopted Dr. Smith's techniques.

If you were correct in your identification of subject and verb in the preceding sentences. Your markings should look like this:

1. Four <u>instances</u> of staphylococcus infection [were reported] by the nursing staff.
2. Becoming hysterical with fright, the <u>child</u> soon [exhibited] cyanoderma.

127

3:    Three community health <u>agencies</u> [have adopted] Dr. Smith's techniques.

You've probably marked these practice sentences by the standard rules of English grammar. However, you can also think of the subject in sentence 1 as being more than just *instances*. Disregarding all the technicalities of modifiers and the like, you can see *Four instances of staphylococcus infection* as the whole subject. If you marked the sentences that way, you're doing fine. Since we're talking about practical applications of communication skills, why not start thinking of the whole subject of each sentence?

When you look closely at the sentence below, you'll see that it is grammatically correct.

<u>Liver biopsies</u> [showed] the appearance of inflammation, [revealed] degeneration of productive functions, [indicated] development of fibrosis, [uncovered] nodule formation, and [presented] evidence of bile retention.

There is a subject present and also verbs—lots of verbs—so many, in fact, that communication is endangered. The reader might forget what the subject is by the time he reads through all those verbs. It's much better to break up a multiverb sentence like this into several sentences. Remember

FOR THE SAKE OF CLARITY, SENTENCES
SHOULD CONTAIN NO MORE
THAN <u>TWO SUBJECTS</u> AND/OR
<u>TWO VERBS</u>.

Try your hand at straightening out some sentences with too many subjects, too many verbs, or both.

Rewrite the following sentences, to improve their clarity.

1:    A summary of eight experiments appeared in the report, the lecturer presented four more, the lab assignment for the day included six others, and the textbook discussed three more.

2:    Six orderlies, three surgeons, two student nurses, a pathologist, an X-ray technician, and four interns came from their homes, left the lounge, ran from the lab, jumped into the elevator and hurried down the hall.

3:    The physician and the nurse diagnose and treat the patient, and the hospital staff and the paramedical personnel provide support services and hygiene education, while the health worker and the social worker offer consultation and follow-up care in the home environment.

Don't rush. Give these sentences some thought. The objective of this practice is *clarity of communication.*

The preceding sentences could have been rewritten in several different ways. However you rewrote the sentences, you were correct if each rewritten sentence contained no more than *two* subjects and *two* verbs. For example, sentence 1 could have been broken up into two sentences, each containing two subjects and two verbs:

A summary of eight experiments [appeared] in the report, and the lecturer [presented] four more. The lab assignment for the day [included] six others, and the textbook [discussed] three more.

Sentence 2 was thoroughly confused, wasn't it? There was no way to tell who was doing what when. So almost anything you did in the rewriting must have been an improvement. If your rewritten version has no more than two subjects and two verbs per sentence, then you're correct. Here's one way you could have straightened it out:

Six orderlies [came] from their homes as three surgeons [left] the lounge. Two student nurses and a pathologist [ran] from the lab and [jumped] into the elevator. An X-ray technician [hurried] down the hall.

When you studied sentence 3, you probably noticed that it was grammatically correct. But remember: our objective here is *clarity of communication*. So your rewrite should have carved this overly complicated sentence into shorter sentences, none of which contained more than two subjects and two verbs. You could have done this in any of a number of ways. Here's just one possibility:

The physician and the nurse [diagnose] and [treat] the patient. The hospital staff and the paramedical personnel [provide] support services and hygiene education. The health worker and the social worker [offer] consultation and follow-up care in the home environment.

How about it? Did you make clear, meaningful sentences out of those verbal jumbles? Your rewrites may not even resemble those above. But if your sentences contained no more than two subjects and/or two verbs each, then you did a good job. If you still don't feel confident, try the rewriting again.

In taking the pre-test to this unit, you might have had difficulty with some of the sentences that suffered from mismatched word forms. Mismatching word forms in a sentence is an easy mistake to make, but it's one that can get in the way of clear communication.

The following sample sentence contains two verbs—a good number—but the verbs are mismatched in form. When you read it, you can probably get the writer's message, but you might have to look at it twice to be sure. In the health professions, you might not have a chance to look at a message twice. It must be written clearly the first time!

The computer, when used for diagnostic assistance, [requires] no sleep and [is used] day and night.

The clarity difficulty here comes from the mismatching of the verb forms. To rewrite this sentence correctly, you'd need to change the form of one of the verbs. For instance you might change *is used* to *works* so that the verb forms match.

In the following sample sentence, the forms of the objects are mismatched. the objects are enclosed in (parentheses).

Pharmacists usually [prefer] (practicing) privately or (to work) on a hospital staff.

To be clear and correct, this sentence should contain matching object forms. The objects should be either *to practice* and *to work*, or *practicing* and *working*. Remember

> WHEN THEY APPEAR IN THE SAME
> SENTENCE, SUBJECT *MUST MATCH*
> SUBJECT, [VERB] *MUST MATCH*
> [VERB], (OBJECT) *MUST MATCH*
> (OBJECT).

Here are three sentences in which you'll find some mismatching forms. Work carefully in analyzing the errors. Rewrite each sentence so that the word forms match correctly.

1: To learn microbiology and applying it to clinical problems are often quite different things.
2: The physical therapist was prescribing hydrotherapy and called for a strict exercise program.
3: The responsibilities of the health-care team include curing illness and to encourage good health practices.

You probably found most of the preceding practice work to be pretty simple. As usual, there were many ways to rewrite the three sentences. If your rewrites produced sentences in which the forms of subjects matched subjects, the forms of verbs matched verbs, and the forms of objects matched objects, then you are correct.

The problem in sentence 1 was that the subject forms were mismatched. You could have changed either *to learn* or *applying* and you could have come up with something like this:

Learning microbiology and applying it to clinical problems are often quite different things.

In sentence 2, you probably noticed that the verb forms were mismatched. If your rewrite changed either *was prescribing* or *called*, then you're correct. Here's one way of correcting sentence 2:

The physical therapist [prescribed] hydrotherapy and [called] for a strict exercise program.

The objects were mismatched in sentence 3. In rewriting, you should have changed either *curing* or *to encourage*. You may have written something like this:

> The responsibilities of the health-care team include (curing) illness and (encouraging) good health practices.

If you're still not certain about the matching of word forms within the sentence, repeat this practice cycle again.

This is the last communication practice exercise in this unit, but it's one that gives everybody trouble at some time or other. So look at it carefully.

Remember this sentence from the pre-test?

> Megalomania is not an attribute of a good physician and can lead them to expect unattainable successes.

The problem here, of course, is that the word *physician* is singular, but the pronoun that refers to it, *them*, is plural. To be correct, *them* should be *him*. In a way, this is another case of mismatched forms. But this is a particular kind of situation. Always be careful to match singular forms with singular forms and plural forms with plural forms. Or, to put it another way

> WORDS THAT RELATE TO ONE ANOTHER
> MUST BE ALIKE IN EITHER *SINGULAR*
> OR *PLURAL* FORM.

Take a look at the following sample sentence and see how the singular and plural forms are *correctly* matched:

> A nurse, because of overcrowding and understaffing in the hospital, often cares for too many patients.

In this sentence, the words *nurse* and *cares* are correctly matched, right? They are both plural forms. But in this sentence—

> The medical technologist give very important service to the health-care team in any community.

—the subject, *medical technologist*, and the verb, *give*, are not correctly matched. In this case, the best correction would be to add an *s* to *give* in order to make it match the singular form of *medical technologist*.

Now read the following sentences carefully and find out where the singular/plural errors appear. Then rewrite each sentence correctly.

1: Although uvulas are peculiar looking, it does play an important part in pronunciation.

2:   The RBC, one of the lab technician's most frequent tasks, are important tools in diagnostic work.

3:   Chronic complaints of gastralgia sometimes indicates a prescription of Alka-Seltzer and relaxation.

4:   Dentists frequently attributes the patient's lack of attention to oral hygiene with many of their dental disorders.

Check your rewrites carefully until you're sure you've found and corrected all the errors then continue.

Sentence 1 was incorrect because the forms of *uvulas* and *it* were mismatched. Any rewrite which put that error back in shape would have been correct. Here's one example:

Although uvulas are peculiar looking, they do play an important part in pronunciation.

There was a serious mistake in the matching of the subject, *RBC*, and the verb, *are*, in sentence 2. You're correct if you changed the verb to match the subject. You should also have changed the plural form of *tools* to match the singular subject form. Your rewrite might look something like this:

The RBC, one of the lab technician's most frequent tasks, is an important tool in diagnostic work.

Sentence 3 also contained mismatched subject and verb forms. Did you catch them? You could have changed either form to make it match the other. This is one way to rewrite sentence 3:

Chronic complaints of gastralgia sometimes indicate prescriptions of Alka-Seltzer and relaxation.

Sentence 4 contained a couple of mismatchings, and you should have caught and corrected both of them. *Dentists* and *attributes* don't work together, and neither do *patient's* and *their*. (You know that *their* relates to *patient's*, don't you? After all, who's most likely to have dental disorders here?) You could have cleaned up sentence 4 by writing:

Dentists frequently attribute the patient's lack of attention to oral hygiene with many of his dental disorders.

If you're still not comfortable with some of the suggestions for maintaining communication clarity that you've learned here, take a few minutes and work through some sections of this unit. The important thing is how well you've learned, not how long it takes.

You have completed Unit 1. Look over your work carefully.

Review Test for Unit 1

Directions: Like all other review tests in this program, this one is for your use only in checking your learning progress. This is *not* a test to be graded. In each of the following sentences, there are grammatical errors or misconstructions that impair communication clarity. Rewrite it to correct the difficulty or difficulties in the sentence.

1: The patient, still dressed in his examining gown, run through the halls of the clinic.

2: To be able to make a swift, accurate diagnosis and immediately beginning treatment are necessary elements of good emergency room practice.

3: Making a proper dental impression is at least as important as to properly use dental examining tools.

4: Lack of attention to such physical symptoms as cyanoderma have resulted in tragic consequences.

5: Taking readings of pulse and blood pressure, measuring weight and height, recording parts or family and personal histories, and running fundamental blood tests and urinalyses are functions of the physician's nurse.

6: Dr. Howard's research demonstrated the interaction of certain enzymes, revealed previously unknown properties of gastric acids, explored the significance of gastroduodenal carcinoma, and supported earlier research in the field of gastrology.

7: Encouraging patients, administering medications, directing the staff and reporting to doctors demands the time, frays and nerves, tests the patience, tries the imagination, and shapes the character of the nurse.

8: All health professionals should understand the compounding of chemicals and how to use drugs properly.

9: The crucial need for health practitioners in disadvantaged communities grow every day.

10: A health science student's ability to observe precisely and objectively will be of value to them throughout their professional life.

You have completed Review Test 1. Look over your work carefully. When you feel that you have done your best, check your work with the answers. Correct any incorrect answers, but mark them for future reference.

ANSWERS: UNIT 1

1. The error is the disagreement between *patient* and *run*. You should have changed the sentence to correct this mismatching. Here's one way in which you could have rewritten it:
   The patient, still dressed in his examining gown, ran through the halls of the clinic.

2. There is mismatching between *to be able to make* and *beginning*. Any rewrite that correctly matched the forms would be correct.

3. The error here is the same as in sentence 2: a mismatching between the forms of *making* and *to . . . use*. Your rewrite should match the two forms of these two subjects correctly.

4. *Lack of attention* and *have* are mismatched. A correct rewrite would probably change *have* to *has*.

5. In this sentence, there are too many subjects. If you broke this long sentence into several shorter ones—each with no more than two subjects—then you're correct.

6. Sentence 6 contains too many verbs. As in sentence 5, you should break this sentence into several shorter ones, none with more than two verbs.

7. Here there are too many subjects and too many verbs. Your rewrite should break this sentence up into several shorter sentences. Each sentence should have no more than two subjects and two verbs.

8. Here's another sample of mismatching. *Compounding* and *how to use* are both objects, so they should have matched forms. If you changed either one to match the form of the other, you were correct.

9. The subject here is *need* and the verb is *grow*. You probably saw that the two forms don't match. Your rewrite should change one to match the form of the other.

10. If you studied this one carefully, you saw that *them* and *their* are plural, whereas *student's* is singular. To correct this sentence, you should have changed either *student's* or *them* and *their*. You might have done it this way:

    A health science student's ability to observe precisely and objectively will be of value to him throughout his professional life.

Pre-Test:
Organization Unit 2

Directions: This pre-test is designed to measure your present ability to (1) recognize and mark the organizational elements of a paragraph and (2) organize a series of statements into a well-ordered and expressive paragraph. Please *do not* change any of your work after checking the answers.

Use the indicated symbols to mark the organizational elements of the following paragraph.

1. Underline all subject sentences.
2. Place [brackets] around each sentence of exposition.
3. Place (parentheses) around each sentence of conclusion.
4. Place ⟨diamond brackets⟩ around each transitional phrase.

The team concept in health-care delivery is only now becoming acceptable to many health professionals. It calls for all persons involved in the health care in a given community to recognize the interdependence of various professional roles. Today, the physician, the dentist, the nurse, the therapist, the public health professional, and others need to work together in order to provide the most comprehensive health care. Without this integrated team approach, it is likely that the community's total health needs will go unmet.

Organize the following series of statements into a carefully ordered paragraph.

1: So, the nature of renal involvement is becoming more clearly understood.
2: Many cases have been reported in the literature, and the clinical features of nephropathy have been fully dscribed.
3: Renal involvement in secondary syphilis has been recognized for at least 150 years.
4: The development of renal biopsy has contributed further to the understanding of this condition.
5: It was first hypothesized in 1825.

PRE-TEST ANSWERS

If you marked the first paragraph correctly, it should look like this:

The team concept in health-care delivery is only now becoming acceptable to many health professionals. [It calls for all persons involved in the health care of a given community to recognize the interdependence of various professional roles.] [Today, the physician, the dentist, the nurse, the therapist, the public health professional, and others need to work together in order to provide the most comprehensive health care.] (Without this integrated team approach, it is likely that the community's total health needs will go unmet.)

If you correctly organized the series of statements, your paragraph should read like this:

Renal involvement in secondary syphilis has been recognized for at least 150 years. It was first hypothesized in 1825. Many cases have been reported in the literature, and the clinical features of nephropathy have been fully described. The development of renal biopsy has contributed further to the understanding of this condition. So, the nature of renal involvement is becoming more clearly understood.

You have completed this pre-test. Please do not change any of your work. If your work was 100 percent correct, skip to the pre-test to Unit 3; if less than 100 percent correct, proceed to Unit 2.

UNIT 2

For all practical purposes, the sentence is the basic unit of communication. In each sentence, there is at least one subject and one verb. The purpose of the subject is to name the person, place, or thing that the sentence is about. The purpose of the verb is to define or describe the subject in some detail.

Look at the following sentence:

Arthritis [disrupts] the movements of affected joints.

The subject of the sentence, what it's about, is arthritis. The verb, [disrupts], defines or describes arthritis in some detail. If the sentence contains a compound verb, the subject is defined or described in greater detail:

Arthritis [disrupts] the movements of affected joints and [produces] painful tissue swelling.

Now you know that arthritis not only [disrupts], but it [produces], too. Note one other thing about the relationship between the subject and the verbs in this and every sentence:

EVERY VERB RELATES DIRECTLY
TO ITS SUBJECT.

Whether a verb defines or describes; whether it is past, present, or future tense, it sitll must say something specific about its subject.

In the following sentence, the subject, megalocardia, is both defined and described by its verbs. Mark the subject of the sentence with underlining and enclose each verb in brackets [ ].

Megalocardia is a heart condition and can be caused by exercise.

Okay, you've underlined megalocardia and bracketed [is] and [can be caused]. Whether you recognize it or not—and there's no reason why you should—you have just established

137

the relationship between the *subject sentence* and the sentences of *exposition* that exists in a well-organized paragraph. In a paragraph

> THE SUBJECT SENTENCE STATES
> WHAT THE PARAGRAPH IS ABOUT.
> EXPOSITION SENTENCES DEFINE OR
> DESCRIBE THE SUBJECT.

The *paragraph* is structurally similar to the *sentence*. There is a subject in each. And in the paragraph, sentences of exposition—like verbs in a sentence—*define or describe the Subject.*

In the following sentence, bracket the words that define or describe the subject.

> In each experiment, the researcher tested three compounds and conducted biological measurements.

In this sentence, you were correct if you place brackets around [tested] and [ran] —the words that define or describe the subject, <u>researcher</u>.

Now, in the following paragraph, place brackets around each sentence that defines or describes the subject sentence, which is the first one.

> Inoculation against German measles is a standard practice in most American communities today. It is an entrance requirement of many elementary schools. In other areas, it is strongly urged by public health officers.

You were correct if you bracketed the second and third sentences in the paragraph. These two sentences *define or describe* the subject of the paragraph, which is the practice of German measles inoculation in most American communities.

In the following list of statements, select and <u>underline</u> the one which seems to say what all of them are about. Then [bracket] the ones that define or describe the underlined statement.

1: Often the source of drinking water is used for waste disposal and bathing purposes.
2: In some cases, this cycle is maintained for many years.
3: Impure drinking water constitutes a severe health hazard in many underdeveloped countries.
4: Acute bacterial contamination of drinking water causes disease in individuals, who then return the bacteria to the water supply through their waste.

You were correct if you underlined sentence 3 on the preceding page and bracketed sentences 1, 2, and 4. Sentence 3 states the subject of the paragraph—the severe health hazard of impure drinking water. Then, as your probably noticed, each of the other sentences explains, defines, or describes that subject in some way. A sentence that did not refer to the subject would not belong in the paragraph.

IN A PARAGRAPH, EVERY SENTENCE
OF EXPOSITION MUST EXPLAIN,
DEFINE OR DESCRIBE THE SUBJECT
IN SOME WAY.

By now you've probably seen a motive coming clear in all this work: the establishment of an easily remembered, easily applied form for clear, concise organization of information and ideas.

Here's one more bit of practice for you. Study the following list of sentences. Then, in the blanks by the numbers that follow, rearrange these sentences. Put the subject sentence first; then follow it with the other sentences of exposition in what seems like the best order.

1:    Three interns came running down the hall.
2:    A nurse leaped from the elevator.
3:    Six people hurried to answer the emergency room call.
4:    After them ran a pathologist and two surgeons.

Now, rearrange them here:

1.   _____
2.   _____
3.   _____
4.   _____

Look carefully at your arrangement. Be sure you know why you put each sentence where you did.

You should have rearranged the sentences like this:

1.   Six people hurried to answer the emergency room call.
2.   A nurse leaped from the elevator.
3.   Three interns came running down the hall.
4.   After them ran a pathologist and two surgeons.

Of course, it's easy to see the content relationship among these four sentences. And that relationship is best expressed in the sentence which should be the first one in your list. In a paragraph, then, the sentence "Six people hurried to answer the emergency room call" would be a good choice as the subject sentence.

The other three sentences actually describe the subject in greater detail. Consequently, each of these three sentences qualifies as a sentence of exposition.

To extend this idea to its conclusion, you had to look carefully at the wording of each sentence. In their original order, either sentence 1 or 2 could follow sentence 3, the subject sentence. But sentence 4, with the words "after them," could only follow sentence 1. So you're probably safe if you arranged the sentences in the order suggested at the top of this page.

A CLEAR, WELL-ORGANIZED PARAGRAPH
CONTAINS A <u>SUBJECT</u> SENTENCE
AND SEVERAL SENTENCES OF
<u>EXPOSITION</u>.

The third major element in a well-organized paragraph is the *conclusion*. The conclusion restates, wraps up, or in some other way completes the paragraph's presentation of ideas or information. Look carefully at the following paragraph:

> <u>The process of diagnosing a patient's complaint is usually very involved.</u> [A physical examination is often required.] [The patient's personal and family health histories must be taken.] [Laboratory tests sometimes prove necessary.] (If the physician is to be sure of his diagnosis, he must go through all the proper steps.)

In this paragraph, you recognize the subject sentence and the sentences of exposition by the symbols that mark them. The last sentence in the paragraph is the conclusion, marked with parentheses. It restates, in somewhat different words, the idea of the subject sentence.

Read the following paragraph very carefully. Then <u>underline</u> the subject sentence, [bracket] the exposition sentences, and place (parentheses) around the conclusion.

> Bacteriology is an important area of health sciences research. Since man first discovered that most disease is transmitted by minute organisms, the study of bacteria has grown more complex. Bacteriologists are now benefiting all health science with their findings on the pathogenic role of viruses. It is difficult to overstate the importance of bacteriological investigative efforts.

If you read the paragraph carefully, you probably underlined the first sentence as the subject sentence. Brackets should have been placed around the second and third sentences, as exposition. The last sentence, the conclusion, should have been marked with parentheses.

Note how each of the exposition sentences and the conclusion seem to support the subject sentence. The exposition sentences define or describe the subject of the paragraph. The conclusion restates or otherwise completes the paragraph's presentation of the subject.

IN A WELL-ORGANIZED PARAGRAPH,
THE <u>CONCLUSION</u> RESTATES
OR OTHERWISE COMPLETES THE <u>SUBJECT</u>
OF THE PARAGRAPH.

Study the following list of sentences carefully. Then mark the subject sentence with an <u>underline</u>, [bracket] the sentences of exposition, and place (parentheses) around the conclusion.

1: The transplanting of kidneys is almost an everyday event in United States hospitals.

2: With each successful operation, organ transplantation becomes a more refined and hazard-free procedure.

3: Corneal transplants have proved extremely successful.

4: The replacement of damaged or diseased organs with transplanted ones is no longer a mysterious or experimental operation.

5: Soon, perhaps, even entire body systems can be transplanted successfully.

Now write the appropriate sentence number in the blank by the name of each organizational element.

Subject sentence: _____

Exposition 1: _____   Exposition 3: _____

Exposition 2: _____   Conclusion: _____

Your work should look something like this:

1. [The transplanting of kidneys is almost an everyday event in United States hospitals.]

2. [With each successful operation, organ transplantation becomes a more refined and hazard-free procedure.]

3. [Corneal transplants haved proved extremely successful.]

4. <u>The replacement of damaged or diseased organs with transplanted ones is no longer a mysterious or experimental procedure.</u>

5. (Soon, perhaps, even entire body systems can be transplanted successfully.)

As is usually the case, you're left with a wide range of choice in arranging the sentences in order. The placement of the subject and the conclusion is pretty obvious, of course, but you can be rather free with the order of the exposition sentences. Here's an order that looked good to me. How does it check with yours?

Subject sentence: 4

Exposition 1:   1   Exposition 3:   2

Exposition 2:   3   Conclusion: 5

Now take another look at the preceding sentence–arranging exercise. What you have done here is to build a *basic outline for the organization of a paragraph.*

Subject Sentence
Exposition 1
Exposition 2
Exposition 3
Conclusion

If you keep in mind this simple outline and a few rules of relationships, you should have little difficulty writing well-organized sentences and well-organized paragraphs.

EVERY SENTENCE NEEDS A SUBJECT
AND AN EXPOSITION. EVERY PARAGRAPH
NEEDS A SUBJECT AND EXPOSITION.
EXPOSITIONS MUST BE RELATED
DIRECTLY TO THE SUBJECTS.

Since you've learned to identify and organize sentences expressing the subject, exposition, and conclusion of a paragraph, you'll enjoy the opportunity to build a paragraph from the ground up. Each of the following informational phrases and word groups is related in content to all the others. Construct an organized sentence from each one. Then order your new sentences and combine them into a well-organized paragraph. You'll need to "make up" a concluding sentence, of course, since the conclusion is a restatement of the major ideas in the paragraph. Here's the list:

1:    *lymphatic carcinoma fastest spreading type*
2:    *lymph system serves whole body*
3:    *matter of weeks*
4:    *cancer advances different rates*
5:    *tissue with slow exchange rate with body not as dangerous*
6:    *breast cancer rather slow growth*
7:    *early detection beneficial all cases*

Of course, you have made your own word choices and syntactical arrangements in building the preceding sentences. The sentences below reflect my own choices, which are not necessarily any better than yours. But the order of the sentences in the final paragraph is probably as nearly "correct" as anything of this sort can be.

1.   *lymphatic carcinoma fastest spreading type*
       The subject of this sentence is clear, but there is no exposition (verb). When I added exposition to define or describe the subject, I come up with
       [Lymphatic carcinoma is the fastest spreading type of cancer.]

2:    *lymph system serves whole body*
       Both the subject and the exposition (verb) are present. I added a few words to fill out the sentence.
       [The lymph system serves the whole body.]

3.   *matter of weeks*
       Although an idea is suggested here, there is neither subject nor exposition in these words. So I took a couple of cues from the content of the other word groups and wrote
       [It can spread cancer throughout the body in a matter of weeks.]

4.   *cancer advances different rates*
       Again, the subject and exposition are both present, so you only needed to fill in a few words. I chose these:
       Cancer advances through body tissue at varying rates of growth.

5. *tissue with slow exchange rate with body not as dangerous*
   A subject and a nearly complete idea are present, but a definite exposition is needed. I also added a few words to fill out the sentence.
   [Tissue with a slow rate of exchange with the rest of the body does not spread cancerous cells as dangerously fast.]

6. *breast cancer rather slow growth*
   The addition of exposition (a verb) and some other words gave me
   [Breast cancer, for example, exhibits rather slow growth.]

7. *early detection beneficial all cases*
   I inserted a word of exposition and filled out the sentence.
   (But early detection is beneficial to the treatment of all cancer cases.)

   Then, with the sentences organized and marked, I wrote my paragraph as you see it below. Again, you may have made different choices in organizing your paragraph. As long as your organization is logical internally, that's fine.

> *Cancer advances through body tissue at varying rates of growth. Lymphatic carcinoma is the fastest spreading type of cancer. The lymph system serves the whole body. It can spread cancer throughout the body in a matter of weeks. Tissue with a slow rate of exchange with the rest of the body does not spread cancerous cells as dangerously fast. Breast cancer, for example, exhibits rather slow growth. But early detection is beneficial to the treatment of all cancer cases.*

If your organizational patterns differ markedly from the preceding paragraph, maybe you'd better recheck your work and look back over the last few exercises.

You have completed Unit 2. Look over your work in this unit carefully.

Pre-Test:
Organization Unit 3

Directions: This pre-test, like all others in this program, is designed to measure your skills at this point. Complete as much of the work as possible. Then check your work. Please *do not* change any of your pre-test work after checking the answers.

Prepare an outline model for a five-paragraph paper, using the subject/exposition/conclusion format that you learned in Unit 2.

PRE-TEST ANSWERS

The outline model for a five-paragraph paper should look like this:

Subject Sentence

A

B

C

Conclusion

Sentence A

a-1

a-2

a-3

a-conclusion

Sentence B

b-1

b-2

b-3

b-conclusion

Sentence C

c-1

c-2

c-3

c-conclusion

Conclusion

conclusion-1-conclusion

If your work on this pre-test was 100 percent correct, you are finished; if *less* than 100 percent correct, proceed to Unit 3.

UNIT 3

First, let's try a quick review. Read the following sentence and mark it for subject and [exposition].

In the past 100 years, three great actions have profoundly altered the education of our national human resources.

Now read the following paragraph and mark it for subject, exposition, and conclusion.

In the past 100 years, three great actions have profoundly altered the education of our national human resources. The Abolition of Slavery introduced into American society the concept of educational, as well as social and legal, equality for every sector of the citizenry. The Morrill Act of 1862 established the precedent of national aid to education in the form of land-grant colleges. In 1965–66, Congress passed Medicare and Medicaid legislation, which changed the concept of health care from an individual to a social responsibility and presented new challenges to medical education. The changes ordered in our social structure by these three momentous actions demand a review of our educational methods and goals.

Now let's check it to be sure that you haven't forgotten the details of what you learned in Units 1 and 2. In the sentence, you should have marked three great actions as the subject and either [altered] or the rest of the sentence as the exposition.

The paragraph is in order, with the first sentence as the subject, the next three sentences as exposition, and the final sentence as the conclusion. If you marked all these elements, then you're ready to proceed.

Please note in the preceding paragraph that sentences 2, 3, and 4 all define, describe, or explain sentence 1, the subject. The subject sentence names three great actions. The next three sentences tell you what those actions were. Then the conclusion wraps up the paragraph with a subtle rephrasing of the subject. In outline form, the paragraph looks like this:

Subject sentence
Exposition A
Exposition B
Exposition C
Conclusion

You've probably noticed that the preceding outline form could be expanded a little and used to develop a multiple-paragraph paper. This would work because a paper or report should contain the same elements—in a different form—that you've learned to use in writing a well-organized paragraph. To put it more strongly,

> EVERY MULTIPLE-PARAGRAPH PAPER SHOULD HAVE A SUBJECT PARAGRAPH, SEVERAL PARA-GRAPHS OF EXPOSITION AND A PARAGRAPH OF CONCLUSION.

Here's how that outline might look if you expanded it to develop a three-paragraph paper or report:

	Subject Sentence
	Exposition A
Subject	*Exposition B*
	Exposition C
	Conclusion
	Subject Sentence
	Exposition
Exposition	*Exposition*
	Exposition
	Conclusion
	Subject Sentence
	Exposition
Conclusion	*Exposition*
	Exposition
	Conclusion

Now try your hand at sketching the same sort of model outline form. Build one for a four-paragraph paper or report.

Your model outline form should be very similar to the one that I showed you, except that your model should have four exposition paragraphs instead of three.

Read the following five-paragraph paper very carefully. As you do, (1) make notes in the margin to indicate the paragraphs of subject, exposition, and conclusion, and (2) watch for any peculiarities that may crop up.

In the past 100 years, three great actions have profoundly altered the education of our national human resources. The Abolition of Slavery introduced into American society the concept of educational, as well as social and legal, equality for every sector of the citizenry. The Morrill Act of 1862 established the precedent of national aid to education in the form of land-grant colleges. In 1965–66, Congress passed Medicare and Medicaid legislation, which changed the concept of health care from an individual to a social responsibility. The changes in our social structure ordered by these three momentous actions demand a review of our educational methods and goals.

The Abolition of Slavery introduced into American society the concept of educational, as well as social and legal, equality for every sector of the citizenry. Although this concept faced prolonged resistance, the mid-twentieth century finds full educational opportunity for minority groups coming belatedly but profoundly to realization. Postgraduate institutions are opening their doors and expanding their curricula to meet the needs of minority-group students. Minority segments of society are beginning to feel the impact of increasing numbers of trained professionals who return to practice in their home communities. The hopes of the relatively few men who a century ago began planning for the total welfare of man are being bolstered daily.

The Morrill Act of 1862 established the precedent of national aid to education in the form of land-grant colleges. The Act orginally called only for the building of agricultural colleges. But since 1890, those agricultural colleges have become some of the nation's strongest universities. Senator Morrill's initial conception of federally underwritten higher education has made learning available to millions whose potential for humane service might otherwise have been stifled.

In 1965–66, Congress passed Medicare and Medicaid legislation, which changed the concept of health care from an individual to a social responsibility. With the establishment of a national tax basis for medical care, such care has become the human right of every citizen. The medical profession and particularly medical educators are challenged to accept more responsibility for structuring the health-maintenance organization of the future. We must all cooperate to assure society of competent health care for all its members.

The changes in our social structure ordered by these three momentous actions demand a review of our educational methods and goals. This is the only way in which the challenges of history and the needs of humanity can be met.

If you saw the five-paragraph essay in the same way that I did, you probably marked the first paragraph as the subject paragraph, the next three paragraphs as exposition, and the last paragraph as conclusion.

You may have noticed, too, that one of the peculiarities that cropped up was the repetition of certain sentences. In fact, every one of the sentences in the subject paragraph was repeated later in the paper. Look back at the essay and observe *where* those sentences were repeated.

Each exposition sentence in the first paragraph became a subject sentence in one of the later exposition paragraphs. If that's a little confusing, look at it in outline form:

> *Subject Sentence*
> > *Exposition A*
> > *Exposition B*
> > *Exposition C*
> *Conclusion*
>
> *Subject sentence A*
> > *Exposition a-1*
> > *Exposition a-2*
> > *Exposition a-3*
> *Conclusion a*
>
> *Subject Sentence B*
> > *Exposition b-1*
> > *Exposition b-2*
> > *Exposition b-3*
> *Conclusion b*
>
> *Subject Sentence C*
> > *Exposition c-1*
> > *Exposition c-2*
> > *Exposition c-3*
> *Conclusion c*
>
> *Subject Sentence—conclusion*
> > *conclusion- 1- conclusion*

After studying the outline carefully, draw connecting lines from each exposition sentence in the first paragraph of the essay to its place as a subject sentence in a following paragraph.

Without looking back, complete the following outline for a five-paragraph paper.

Paragraph 1:   *Subject sentence*
> > *Exposition A*
> > *Exposition B*
> > *Exposition C*
> *Conclusion*

Paragraph 2:

Paragraph 3:

Paragraph 4:

Paragraph 5:

To check your work, refer back to the outline model.

For your final practice exercise in this unit, write a four-paragraph paper. Use the following paragraph as your subject paragraph, and follow as closely as possible the outline model that you just learned. Use details from any source, or make them up. The emphasis here is on the proper form, not on content.

> *The scope and aims of allied health services have expanded radically in the past 10 years. Once, there were few professional areas in what is now called allied health. Today, however, allied health professionals provide a wide variety of necessary and unique health care services. Allied health is a continually growing professional field.*

There is no way for me to know exactly what you wrote for exposition paragraphs. However, your multiple-paragraph form is essentially correct if it looks like this:

Paragraph 1:
> *The scope and aims of allied health services have expanded radically in the past ten years.*
>> (Discuss briefly how health services have broadened in coverage, etc.)

Paragraph 2:

Once, there were few professional areas in what is now called allied health.

(Continue your exposition with brief remarks on old ways.)

Paragraph 3:

Today, however, allied health professionals provide a wide variety of necessary and unique health care services.

(Discuss several of those new and/or improved health services.)

Paragraph 4:

Allied health is a continually growing professional field.

(Conclude your exposition by listing the opportunities and increasing development of programs, etc.)

As you see, if you organized your paper according to the outline model that you've learned in this unit, there is a strong sense of continuity and cohesiveness running through all paragraphs of your paper. Every paragraph in the paper is well organized and every sentence in the paper relates directly to the overall subject of the paper. This is the objective in clear, well-organized written and spoken communication.

Look back over this unit carefully. Review this outline model on pages 148 and 150. When you have mastered this model, you won't need to repeat the Exposition sentences A, B, C, etc., word for word in the succeeding paragraphs of your paper; that kind of repetition is only used as a learning exercise in this unit. But you should stick with the organizational form that you have established in this unit. It will be of real use to you throughout your health sciences education!

You have completed Unit 3. Look over your work carefully to be sure you are satisfied with it.